ENHANCING THE VITALITY OF THE NATIONAL INSTITUTES OF HEALTH

ORGANIZATIONAL CHANGE TO MEET NEW CHALLENGES

Committee on the Organizational Structure of the
National Institutes of Health

Board on Life Sciences
National Research Council

Health Sciences Policy Board
Institute of Medicine

NATIONAL RESEARCH COUNCIL
INSTITUTE OF MEDICINE
OF THE NATIONAL ACADEMIES

THE NATIONAL ACADEMIES PRESS
Washington, D.C.
www.nap.edu

THE NATIONAL ACADEMIES PRESS   500 Fifth Street, N.W.   Washington, DC 20001

NOTICE: The project that is the subject of this report was approved by the Governing Board of the National Research Council, whose members are drawn from the councils of the National Academy of Sciences, the National Academy of Engineering, and the Institute of Medicine. The members of the committee responsible for the report were chosen for their special competences and with regard for appropriate balance.

This study was supported by Contract/Grant No. N01-OD-4-2139 between the National Academy of Sciences and the National Institutes of Health. Any opinions, findings, conclusions, or recommendations expressed in this publication are those of the author(s) and do not necessarily reflect the views of the organizations or agencies that provided support for the project.

International Standard Book Number 0-309-08967-0 (Book)
International Standard Book Number 0-309-52573-X (PDF)

Library of Congress Conrol Number 2003113301

Additional copies of this report are available from the National Academies Press, 500 Fifth Street, N.W., Lockbox 285, Washington, DC 20055; (800) 624-6242 or (202) 334-3313 (in the Washington metropolitan area); Internet, http://www.nap.edu

Copyright 2003 by the National Academy of Sciences. All rights reserved.

Printed in the United States of America

THE NATIONAL ACADEMIES
Advisers to the Nation on Science, Engineering, and Medicine

The **National Academy of Sciences** is a private, nonprofit, self-perpetuating society of distinguished scholars engaged in scientific and engineering research, dedicated to the furtherance of science and technology and to their use for the general welfare. Upon the authority of the charter granted to it by the Congress in 1863, the Academy has a mandate that requires it to advise the federal government on scientific and technical matters. Dr. Bruce M. Alberts is president of the National Academy of Sciences.

The **National Academy of Engineering** was established in 1964, under the charter of the National Academy of Sciences, as a parallel organization of outstanding engineers. It is autonomous in its administration and in the selection of its members, sharing with the National Academy of Sciences the responsibility for advising the federal government. The National Academy of Engineering also sponsors engineering programs aimed at meeting national needs, encourages education and research, and recognizes the superior achievements of engineers. Dr. Wm. A. Wulf is president of the National Academy of Engineering.

The **Institute of Medicine** was established in 1970 by the National Academy of Sciences to secure the services of eminent members of appropriate professions in the examination of policy matters pertaining to the health of the public. The Institute acts under the responsibility given to the National Academy of Sciences by its congressional charter to be an adviser to the federal government and, upon its own initiative, to identify issues of medical care, research, and education. Dr. Harvey V. Fineberg is president of the Institute of Medicine.

The **National Research Council** was organized by the National Academy of Sciences in 1916 to associate the broad community of science and technology with the Academy's purposes of furthering knowledge and advising the federal government. Functioning in accordance with general policies determined by the Academy, the Council has become the principal operating agency of both the National Academy of Sciences and the National Academy of Engineering in providing services to the government, the public, and the scientific and engineering communities. The Council is administered jointly by both Academies and the Institute of Medicine. Dr. Bruce M. Alberts and Dr. Wm. A. Wulf are chair and vice chair, respectively, of the National Research Council.

www.national-academies.org

COMMITTEE ON THE ORGANIZATIONAL STRUCTURE OF THE NATIONAL INSTITUTES OF HEALTH

HAROLD T. SHAPIRO, *Chair*, Princeton University, Princeton, New Jersey
NORMAN R. AUGUSTINE, Lockheed Martin Corporation, Bethesda, Maryland
J. MICHAEL BISHOP, University of California, San Francisco, California
JAMES R. GAVIN III, Morehouse School of Medicine, Atlanta, Georgia
ALFRED G. GILMAN, University of Texas Southwestern Medical Center, Dallas, Texas
MARTHA N. HILL, Johns Hopkins University School of Nursing, Baltimore, Maryland
DEBRA R. LAPPIN, Princeton Partners Ltd., Denver, Colorado
ALAN I. LESHNER, American Association for the Advancement of Science, Washington, DC
GILBERT S. OMENN, University of Michigan, Ann Arbor, Michigan
FRANKLYN G. PRENDERGAST, Mayo Clinic Cancer Center, Rochester, Minnesota
STEPHEN J. RYAN, University of Southern California, Los Angeles, California
SAMUEL C. SILVERSTEIN, Columbia University College of Physicians and Surgeons, New York, New York
HAROLD C. SLAVKIN, University of Southern California, Los Angeles, California
JUDITH L. SWAIN, Stanford University School of Medicine, Stanford, California
LYDIA VILLA-KOMAROFF, Whitehead Institute, Cambridge, Massachusetts
ROBERT H. WATERMAN, Waterman Group, Inc., Hillsborough, California
MYRL WEINBERG, National Health Council, Washington, DC
KENNETH B. WELLS, University of California, Los Angeles, California
MARY WOOLLEY, Research!America, Alexandria, Virginia
JAMES B. WYNGAARDEN, Duke University, Durham, North Carolina
TADATAKA YAMADA, GlaxoSmithKline, King of Prussia, Pennsylvania

Staff

FRANCES E. SHARPLES, Study Director, Board on Life Sciences, Division on Earth and Life Studies (DELS)
FREDERICK J. MANNING, Senior Program Officer, Board on Health Sciences Policy, Institute of Medicine
ROBIN A. SCHOEN, Senior Program Officer, Board on Life Sciences, DELS
JOAN ESNAYRA, Program Officer, Policy and Global Affairs Division
BRIDGET K. B. AVILA, Senior Project Assistant, Board on Life Sciences, DELS
LYNN CARLETON, Research Intern, Board on Life Sciences, DELS
KATHI E. HANNA, Writer
NORMAN GROSSBLATT, Senior Editor, DELS

BOARD ON LIFE SCIENCES

COREY S. GOODMAN, *Chair*, Renovis, Inc., South San Francisco, California
R. ALTA CHARO, University of Wisconsin, Madison, Wisconsin
JOANNE CHORY, The Salk Institute for Biological Studies, La Jolla, California
JEFFREY L. DANGL, University of North Carolina, Chapel Hill, North Carolina
PAUL R. EHRLICH, Stanford University, Stanford, California
DAVID J. GALAS, Keck Graduate Institute of Applied Life Science, Claremont, California
BARBARA GASTEL, Texas A&M University, College Station, Texas
JAMES M. GENTILE, Hope College, Holland, Michigan
LINDA GREER, Natural Resources Defense Council, Washington, DC
ED HARLOW, Harvard Medical School, Cambridge, Massachusetts
KENNETH F. KELLER, University of Minnesota, Minneapolis, Minnesota
GREGORY A. PETSKO, Brandeis University, Waltham, Massachusetts
STUART L. PIMM, Duke University, Durham, North Carolina
JOAN B. ROSE, Michigan State University, East Lansing, Michigan
GERALD M. RUBIN, Howard Hughes Biomedical Research, Chevy Chase, Maryland
BARBARA A. SCHAAL, Washington University, St. Louis, Missouri
RAYMOND L. WHITE, University of California, San Francisco, California

Staff

FRANCES E. SHARPLES, Director
ROBIN A. SCHOEN, Senior Program Officer
ROBERT T. YUAN, Senior Program Officer
KERRY A. BRENNER, Program Officer
MARILEE K. SHELTON-DAVENPORT, Program Officer
EVONNE P. Y. TANG, Program Officer
BRIDGET K. B. AVILA, Senior Project Assistant
DENISE GROSSHANS, Senior Project Assistant
LYNN CARLETON, Project Assistant/Research Intern
BHAVIT SHETH, Project Assistant
SETH STRONGIN, Project Assistant

Preface

The strong system of federal support for US science and technology has produced five decades of discovery and innovation that have not only literally changed the way we live, but deepened our understanding of the human condition, of our position in the universe, and of our relationship to other forms of life. This use of public resources is widely agreed to have yielded great social dividends for the citizens of our country and beyond. In many ways, the National Institutes of Health (NIH) is unsurpassed among the array of federal agencies that support scientific research, providing 80% of the federal government's contribution to biomedical research. From a humble beginning in the late 19th century as a one room laboratory with a $300 government allocation, NIH has grown into a $27 billion per year organization that justifiably enjoys enormous public and congressional support. NIH's success in its mission of science in pursuit of fundamental knowledge and the application of that knowledge to extending healthy life and reducing the burdens of illness and disability has been enormous. NIH's investment in biomedical research has helped produce remarkable results in terms of declining rates of disease, longer life expectancy, reduced infant mortality, and improved quality of life. All those who have played a role in making NIH such a success over the years have earned the gratitude of current and future generations.

This report was undertaken in response to a congressional request that wisely acknowledged the fact that the world we live in is changing rapidly. In such a world, all enterprises, be they large or small, need to be able to adapt to change if they are to continue to be effective. Indeed in a rapidly changing environment, the greatest risk to successful organizations is the danger of becoming entrenched in the very things that have made them successful at the expense of some needed adaptability. Science and the understanding of health and disease that emerges from science together with an evolving set of health concerns are among the most fast paced areas of change. An organization such as NIH that is dedicated to research and training related to the nation's health concerns must continually consider new ways to meet the challenges of the future. What Congress wants to know is whether NIH's "organizational structure" is right for the times?

As NIH's budget and the number of its organizational units have grown, the complexity of its operations and the ability of its director to manage the overall enterprise have become extremely challenging, especially in light of the loosely federated structure that Congress has established for the NIH. Moreover, all would agree that there surely are some limits to the number and variety of units that any organization's structure, even a loosely federated one, can accommodate. The highly decentralized structure that NIH has evolved over its long history is, in fact, one that most of NIH's constituencies prefer, celebrating the benefits and tolerating the costs of this form of organization. Moreover, these constituencies have often pointed to NIH's obvious success, as if that settled the issue. While NIH's success is to be celebrated, success alone does not answer fully the question of whether there is a better way to proceed, particularly as one faces a future where the world of biomedical science is being rapidly transformed in virtually all its dimensions.

In carrying out its task, our Committee discovered that defining an optimal degree of centralization or decentralization for NIH is not a simple matter. Indeed the right balance between centralization and decentralization is likely to shift over time as circumstances change. The current level of decentralization, together with the institutional relationships among the institutes and centers on the one hand and the study sections and advisory committees on the other, has the great strength of mobilizing a vast array of talent to participate in key decisions. In addition, this mode of operation has the added benefit of helping to secure the support of a large number of constituencies that can point to one or more facets of the organization that reflects their most important concerns. On the other hand, this complex and decentralized organizational structure makes it more difficult for the NIH director to mobilize significant resources to focus on new programs of strategic importance that should engage all the institutes and centers, to support broad based interdisciplinary efforts, and to cooperate in other ways across existing organizational and bureaucratic boundaries.

What became clear to us was that there is no compelling set of management principles that would help either in defining an optimal organizational structure or in identifying the optimal balance between centralization and decentralization for a research organization like NIH, which must not only productively interact with an unusually complex network of constituencies, but also must deal with the inevitable uncertainties and tensions involved in setting a research agenda. In fact, we recognized that the vitality of NIH is only modestly dependent on its formal administrative and organizational structure, but is very dependent on other aspects of the organization's culture and reward system, particularly its capacity to attract and obtain high quality leadership at all levels. In light of such considerations, it was not possible, or useful, to constrain our efforts narrowly to matters that relate purely to NIH's organization chart. While we tried to take a modest approach to our task, the strong and inevitable symbiosis among mission, priorities, and organization meant that we had to consider aspects of all these matters.

In the end, our Committee decided that while the current organizational structure of NIH represents a fundamentally useful response to the legitimate demands made by its varied constituencies, some changes are needed to help NIH meet effectively the new demands of the next decades. While there may be no particular number of institutes and centers that can be shown to be optimal, we came to believe that NIH would be well advised to forge a new set of strategies that could be available to re-deploy some of the efforts of the existing institutes and centers or focus new resources on a revolving set of strategic trans-NIH initiatives that seem compelling. This report presents a variety of ideas identified by the Committee as opportunities for organizational change to improve the agency's responsiveness and flexibility and assist it to continue to accomplish its mission successfully.

Readers of this report should not interpret its recommendations as in any way seeking to undermine the primacy of investigator-initiated science or of the excellent peer review system in place at NIH. The Committee believes that the tens of thousands of NIH-supported scientists working at a couple of thousand institutions must remain the bedrock of NIH's programs. Though not perfect, NIH's peer review system is the best guarantee we have overall that scientists will carry out research that is of high quality and high potential for scientific progress.

I wish to thank all the members of the Committee for their valuable contributions and for their insights into both the scientific and societal issues surrounding this project. The reviewers provided helpful comments that ultimately helped strengthen the report, and I thank them for myself and on behalf of the entire Committee. I also wish to acknowledge the National Academies staff (Fran Sharples, Rick Manning, Robin Schoen, Bridget Avila, and Lynn Carleton) for their thorough and thoughtful assistance with all aspects of the preparation of this report. Joan Esnayra assisted with the pre-study preparations. Kathi Hanna did a superb job in assisting with the writing of the report and was an active participant in many of our discussions. Finally, since we believe the work of NIH to be of ethical significance for both current and future generations, it is our hope that our efforts and our recommendations will stimulate a thoughtful discourse aimed at assisting NIH to move from strength to strength.

Harold T. Shapiro, Chair
Committee on the Organizational Structure of
the National Institutes of Health

Acknowledgments

This report is the product of many individuals. We would like to thank all those people and organizations that provided information and opinions to the committee. A list may be found in Appendix A of this report. Some of the descriptive information in this report was based on a background paper prepared for the National Academies by Michael McGeary and Philip M. Smith. This paper has proved highly useful and we very much appreciate the work done by McGeary and Smith to help get the Committee on the Organizational Structure of the National Institutes of Health off to a good start.

This report has been reviewed in draft form by individuals chosen for their diverse perspectives and technical expertise, in accordance with procedures approved by the National Research Council's Report Review Committee. The purpose of this independent review is to provide candid and critical comments that will assist the institution in making its published report as sound as possible and to ensure that the report meets institutional standards for objectivity, evidence, and responsiveness to the study charge. The review comments and draft manuscript remain confidential to protect the integrity of the deliberative process. We wish to thank the following individuals for their review of this report:

David Baltimore, California Institute of Technology
William G. Barsan, University of Michigan
Arthur I. Bienenstock, Stanford University
Enriqueta C. Bond, Burroughs Wellcome Fund
Charles A. Bowsher, Comptroller General of the United States (former)
Steve Hyman, Harvard University

Richard D. Klausner, The Bill & Melinda Gates Foundation
David Korn, Association of American Medical Colleges
Richard A. Rettig, RAND
Leon E. Rosenberg, Princeton University
Edward M. Scolnick, Merck Research Laboratories
John Seffrin, American Cancer Society
Harold Varmus, Memorial Sloan-Kettering Cancer Center
Raymond White, University of California, San Francisco

Although the reviewers listed above have provided constructive comments and suggestions, they were not asked to endorse the conclusions or recommendations nor did they see the final draft of the report before its release. The review of this report was overseen by Floyd Bloom of The Scripps Research Institute and Mary Jane Osborn of the University of Connecticut Health Center. Appointed by the National Research Council, they were responsible for making certain that an independent examination of this report was carried out in accordance with institutional procedures and that all review comments were carefully considered. Responsibility for the final content of this report rests entirely with the authoring committee and the institution.

Contents

Executive Summary		1
1	Introduction	17
2	The Evolution of NIH'S Organizational Structure	33
3	New Opportunities, New Challenges: The Changing Nature of Biomedical Science	51
4	The Organizational Structure of the National Institutes of Health	67
5	Enhancing NIH's Ability to Respond to New Challenges	83
6	Accountability, Administration, and Leadership	103
7	Putting Principles into Practice	121
References		129
Appendixes		
A	Sources of Information Provided to the Committee	135
B	Acronyms and Abbreviations	139
C	Committee Member Biographies	143

Executive Summary

The continued growth in the number of organizational units of the National Institutes of Health (NIH) has been a cause of both concern and celebration for decades. Numerous NIH officials and external advisory committees have suggested that the continued creation of new units (institutes, centers, and programmatic offices) could impair NIH's functioning by making it unmanageable and impeding its ability to carry out its mission. Most recently, former Director Harold Varmus argued in a 2001 article in *Science* that NIH would be more effective scientifically and more manageable if it were organized into a far smaller number of larger institutes organized around broad areas of science. Others counter that the elimination of units that focus on particular problems would reduce attention to and funding for these problems and that a consolidation of units would reduce congressional and public support and might not be politically feasible. More generally, recent rapid increases in resources, fundamental shifts on the biomedical frontier, and evolving health concerns make it a good moment to review whether the organizational structure of NIH continues to be appropriate.

Clearly many changes have taken place in the world of science and in the nature of the health concerns that research must address. Since the late 1990s, the NIH budget has doubled to its current level of about $27 billion as a result of congressional and presidential initiatives. In science, the importance of multi-institutional, multidisciplinary research that relies more and more on large infrastructural investments is ever more apparent. Demographics and the patterns of illness in society are changing, and the specter of intentional releases of harmful disease organisms by terrorists has emerged following the attacks of September 2001. The private sector's investments in some fields of research have increased to the point where pharmaceutical and biotechnology companies now spend more than NIH on research and development.

With the steady stream of change, concerns about whether NIH has become too fragmented to address effectively the most important biomedical and health challenges or to respond quickly enough to health emergencies have resurfaced in Congress and in some parts of the scientific community. NIH has never been administratively reorganized in any substantial way, only added on to, despite vast changes in the landscape of science and the nation's health concerns during the last half century.

CONGRESSIONAL REQUEST

In report language accompanying the FY 2001 appropriation for the Department of Health and Human Services (DHHS), Congress directed NIH to have the National Academy of Sciences study "whether the current structure and organization of NIH are optimally configured for the scientific needs of the twenty-first century." Senate report 106-293 states:

> The Committee is extremely pleased with the scientific advances that have been made over the past several years due to the Nation's support for biomedical research at NIH. However, the Committee also notes the proliferation of new entities at NIH, raising concerns about coordination. While the Committee continues to have confidence in NIH's ability to fund outstanding research and to ensure that new knowledge will benefit all Americans, the fundamental changes in science that have occurred lead us to question whether the current NIH structure and organization are optimally configured for the scientific needs of the Twenty-first Century. Therefore, the Committee has provided to the NIH Director sufficient funds to undertake, through the National Academy of Sciences, a study of the structure of NIH.

STATEMENT OF TASK

In response to the congressional request, the goal of this study was to determine the optimal NIH organizational structure, given the context of 21st century biomedical research. The following specific questions were to be addressed:

1. Are there general principles by which NIH should be organized?
2. Does the current structure reflect these principles, or should NIH be restructured?
3. If restructuring is recommended, what should the new structure be?
4. How will the proposed new structure improve NIH's ability to conduct biomedical research and training, and accommodate organizational growth in the future?
5. How would the proposed new structure overcome current weaknesses, and what new problems might it introduce?

The Committee on the Organizational Structure of the National Institutes of Health was formed to ensure that the views of the basic science, clinical medicine, and health advocacy communities were all adequately represented. In addition, the committee had members who are experienced in the management of large and complex organizations, including a former NIH director, two former NIH institute directors, a former university president, two persons with backgrounds in senior management of major industrial entities, and a specialist in organizational issues. Several Committee members also had considerable experience in government operations.

The Committee held six two-day meetings over the ten months between July 2002 and April 2003. In its initial meetings it invited past and present representatives of Congress, NIH, voluntary health groups, scientific and professional societies, and industry to provide perspectives on the issues before them (see Appendix A). In addition, the Committee met publicly with the current NIH director as well as several former directors. Committee members and staff also heard presentations from or interviewed NIH staff in the offices of policy and planning, budget, finance, and intramural research, and met with directors of 18 institutes or centers. Data about NIH programs and budgets were requested from NIH staff as the need emerged. Prior reports conducted about and for NIH were reviewed, as was the relevant literature. In addition, the Committee commissioned a background paper tracing the history and evolution of NIH and its institutes as a starting point for its deliberations (McGeary and Smith, 2002). Finally, several Committee members conducted town meetings at their home institutions and elsewhere, inviting scientists, administrators, and students to contribute their perspectives. Thus, the Committee was able to hear, consider, and discuss a diverse range of facts and opinions about the organizational structure of NIH. Its final report and recommendations are, however, based on the Committee's assessment of the information that was available and current trends in biomedical science and health.

THE COMMITTEE'S RESPONSE TO ITS CHARGE

The goal of the study focused on the organizational structure of NIH, but it was not possible to address this issue satisfactorily without considering the mission of NIH, some of its key processes, and the scientific, social, and political environment in which NIH activities take place. Although a long series of reviews of NIH helped to inform committee deliberations, both the nature of the charge and the 1-year period allowed for deliberations put important constraints on the development, character, and scope of the recommendations that could credibly be put forward. Most important, the committee was not asked to address NIH's research priorities or the quality and effectiveness of the wide array of research and advanced training programs that NIH undertakes or sponsors.

The Committee's view of its task was governed, first, by the desire to be of some practical assistance to all those who wish NIH to continue to be an outstanding organization. Scholars of organizational management have long recognized that there is more to organization than structure. An organization's ability to make effective changes is influenced by a multiplicity of factors, including structure, strategy, and systems, the last of which includes all the formal and informal processes and procedures that organizations rely on to function. Thus, the Committee proceeded on the premise that its task included assessing both the organizational configuration of NIH and the key processes and authorities that play roles in NIH-wide decision-making. Although the borders between structure, mission, and priorities are not well defined, the Committee tried not to take too expansive a view of its responsibilities.

Therefore, the Committee did not focus exclusively on whether or not there should be a widespread consolidation of NIH's institutes and centers. Rather, it took a more general approach, namely to inquire if there were any significant organizational changes—including the widespread consolidation of institutes and centers—that would allow NIH to be even more successful in the future. Although the Committee discussed on numerous occasions the advisability of the widespread consolidation of NIH, it eventually came to believe that this was not the best path for NIH to take at this time.

It is important to understand that the structure of any large and complex organization, such as NIH, is not the tidy result of a compact set of compelling propositions emanating from organizational theory any more than the particular organization of our complex pluralistic democracy is the result solely of the inspired thinking of political philosophers. The latter is instead the outcome of our particular form of politics and, therefore, heavily influenced by our history and evolving cultural commitments. It is very much the same way with NIH. It would be naïve to assume that NIH was or should be organized exclusively along the lines dictated either by the interests of the scientific community or the priorities of any other single set of interests with a concern about promoting health-related research and advanced biomedical training. NIH's existing structure is the result of a set of complex evolving social and political negotiations among a variety of constituencies including the Congress, the administration, the scientific community, the health advocacy community, and others interested in research, research training, and public policy related to health. Indeed the history of NIH provides clear evidence that each of these communities has always had a variety of views on the appropriate organization of NIH. From any particular point of view or for any particular set of interests, the current situation is not only imperfect, but is certainly not one that either the Congress or the scientific community would designate *ab initio*. Rather it has evolved as a very useful and largely productive outcome of a series of political and social negotiations that took place over time. This outcome is typical of the design of important social organizations in a pluralistic democracy. NIH has become an organization that balances its many interests and the Committee felt that any major modifications at this point in time should focus directly on enhancing NIH's capacity to pursue major time-limited strategic objectives that cut across all the institutes and to acquire a special ability to pursue more high-risk, high-return projects. It was our view that at this moment the widespread consolidation of institutes and centers is not the next best organizational step for NIH to undertake, as any benefits to be gained would be offset by the costs involved.

What does the Committee mean by "costs"? At a minimum, because Congress created the institutes, dissolving or merging institutes would require congressional action. Any thoughtful major reorganization would necessitate a lengthy and complex information gathering and decision making process that would include numerous congressional hearings involving members of Congress, congressional staff, and a wide variety of interests in the various health advocacy and scientific communities. Our discussions, correspondence, and meetings made it quite clear that there would be very little agreement among these communities on what the right way to reorganize NIH is, and there would probably be dozens of conflicting ideas in play and few clear avenues for narrowing these down. Moreover, these discussions and negotiations would be long and contentious ones and with a quite uncertain outcome. More importantly, the Committee is firmly convinced that many of the goals that might be achieved through large-scale consolidation of institutes could also be achieved more rapidly and effectively through other organizational and administrative mechanisms, as recommended in this report.

Nevertheless the Committee did feel that no organization as important as NIH should remain frozen in organization space and that some regular, thoughtful and publicly transparent mechanism is required to allow appropriate changes in the organizational structure of NIH to take place at appropriate times. Although the Committee does believe that the consolidation of two pairs of institutes is appropriate to consider at this time, it felt that these issues ought to have the benefit of the public process we have recommended.

The Committee was also well aware that all organizational changes, however well thought out, potentially carry both potential risks and benefits, and it has done its best to sort these out. The Committee recognized that the decentralized structure of NIH, which allows a large number of people throughout the scientific and advocacy communities to help to set priorities, has been and should continue to be an integral element in NIH's success. The Committee also kept the enormous benefits of investigator-initiated grants, including those focused on fundamental research, firmly in mind during its deliberations. Finally, the Committee understood that it is the quality of leadership and decision-making at all levels, as opposed to administrative structures, that are central to NIH's vitality. In the long run, the recruitment of outstanding leadership, the commitment to individual scientists as the main sources of new discoveries, and the reliance on the competitive review system for determining awards will be essential to NIH's continuing success.

The fact that NIH has been working well does not mean that it could not work better if—in response to changes on the scientific frontier, new health concerns, or other important environmental shifts—some organizational modifications were made. The intent of this report is to assess the current organizational structure of

NIH and to suggest modifications that might be appropriate to help NIH to become even more effective in supporting research essential to the long-term goal of improving human health.

CENTRALIZATION OF ADMINISTRATIVE FUNCTIONS

NIH is an agency of the Department of Health and Human Services (DHHS), which has recently issued instructions to consolidate administrative functions, such as personnel management, communications, congressional liaison, and travel, throughout the Department. The "One HHS" initiative has the stated goal of better integrating management functions across the department's operating and staff divisions. The initiative has already resulted in consolidation of some administrative functions at NIH. DHHS has further plans for consolidating other functions at NIH, such as budgeting, finance, and procurement, and is encouraging NIH to consider outsourcing some of its administrative functions.

While the Committee believes that it is critical that government continue attempts to eliminate inefficiencies, it would not serve anyone if such initiatives result in decreasing the effectiveness of NIH as a research and training organization or damage its ability to recruit talented leaders at all levels. Centralization of certain functions can be effective, but is not always the best means to achieve increased efficiencies. At times, centralization serves everyone's interests, but at other times it serves no one's interests. The Committee believes that initiatives to centralize or outsource from NIH key science-related functions that are difficult to separate from the performance of its primary mission, such as aspects of grants management, fail to appreciate how closely these administrative functions are tied to the scientific enterprise.

> **Recommendation 1:** *Centralization of Management Functions*
> Any efforts to consolidate or centralize management functions at NIH, either within NIH or at the DHHS level, should be considered only after careful study of circumstances unique to NIH and its successes in carrying out its research and training mission. A structured and studied approach should be used to assure that centralization will not undermine NIH's ability to identify, fund, and manage the best research and training proposals and programs in support of improving health.

ORGANIZATIONAL STRUCTURE OF NIH

NIH's continuing success has been due largely to its ability to adapt to meet the ever-changing needs and challenges posed by science, medicine, and public health. Moreover, there is a perception that given the substantial increases in resources and the vast expansion of the biomedical enterprise, the addition of institutes and centers has been productive and has provided an ever broader base of support and budget success both for the specific interests involved and for NIH in the aggregate. While everyone understands that this expansion cannot and should not continue indefinitely, many see no particular difficulty with the current number of institutes and centers.

The Committee carefully considered major structural changes in NIH, including possible revisions in the number and reporting lines of institutes and centers (ICs) to the director. The Committee considered numerous proposals for restructuring NIH in great detail. However, as laid out in this report, it did not find a compelling intellectual argument for major structural alterations at this time. Rather the Committee makes recommendations for achieving many of the goals identified by proponents of major restructuring (more authority for the NIH director, increased responsiveness, greater flexibility, and more opportunity for coordination) primarily by other means.

Many previous reports have suggested that increasing the number of ICs at NIH would make it less effective. Thus, the present Committee is hardly the first to consider these problems and deliberate over potential solutions. The Committee notes, however, that little changed as a result of past studies. The trend toward continued growth in the number of units in NIH has continued to the present in the absence of an accepted process such as that suggested in the 1984 Institute of Medicine report. The Committee believes therefore that it would be useful for Congress to consider amending the authorizing legislation for NIH to require that certain steps be taken in considering the creation, dissolution, or consolidation of organizational units.

Recommendation 2: *Public Process for Considering Proposed Changes in the Number of NIH Institutes or Centers*
Either on receiving a congressional request or at the discretion of the NIH director in responding to considerable, thoughtful, and sustained interest in changing the number of institutes or centers, the director should initiate a public process to evaluate scientific needs, opportunities, and consequences of the proposed change and the level of public support for it. For a proposed addition, the likelihood of available resources to support it should also be assessed and the burden of proof should reside clearly with those seeking to add an organizational element.

Despite the Committee's conclusion that a large-scale restructuring of the ICs would not be wise now, no organization that is expected to remain effective should have to bear the burden of a frozen organizational structure, and not all its existing units are likely to continue to have the same relevance or independence in the future. Therefore, the public, the scientific community, or the director of NIH, in concert with internal and external advisers, should be able to suggest additions, subtractions, or mergers of units to Congress at appropriate times. The Committee provides two suggestions for potential mergers for further study: the merger of the National

Institute on Drug Abuse and the National Institute on Alcohol Abuse and Alcoholism and the merger of the National Institute of General Medical Sciences and the National Human Genome Research Institute. Indeed, the Committee favors these mergers, but believes that such changes should benefit from use of the process outlined above. However, because of extraordinarily persuasive arguments about exceptional needs made by a variety of groups in discussions with the Committee, it recommends merging several clinical research components of the extramural and intramural programs to create a National Center for Clinical Research & Research Resources.

> Recommendation 3: *Strengthen Clinical Research*
> NIH should pursue a new organizational strategy to better integrate leadership, funding, and management of its clinical research enterprise. The strategy should build on but not replace existing organizational units and activities in the individual ICs' intramural and extramural research programs. It should also include partnerships with the nonprofit and private sectors. Specifically, the Committee recommends that several intramural and extramural programs be combined in a new entity to subsume and replace the National Center for Research Resources, to be called the National Center for Clinical Research and Research Resources (NCCRRR). In addition, a deputy director for clinical research should be appointed in the Office of the Director to serve as deputy director and head of the new entity.

ENHANCING NIH'S ABILITY TO RESPOND TO NEW CHALLENGES

Although the Committee is not recommending a major structural reorganization of NIH's institutes and centers, it concluded that to meet the scientific and health goals of the nation, NIH needs new mechanisms for mobilizing and coordinating funding from many units for high-priority initiatives that cut across the purviews of individual ICs. Although co-funding of projects by multiple institutes occurs, it is not clear to what extent these projects are true "end-to-end" collaborations. Thus, "multi-institute funding" should be distinguished from "trans-NIH initiatives," in which planning and implementation of activities involves more than one institute from start to finish. The Committee believes that the best means to achieve mobilization and coordination of new cross-cutting initiatives is through the initiation via NIH-wide strategic planning of a rotating series of multiyear, but time-limited, strategic initiatives that involve all the ICs.

> Recommendation 4: *Enhance and Increase Trans-NIH Strategic Planning and Funding*
>
> a. The director of NIH should be formally charged by Congress to lead a trans-NIH planning process to identify major crosscutting issues and their associated

research and training opportunities and to generate a small number of major multi-year, but time limited, research programs. The process should be conducted periodically—perhaps every 2 years—and should involve substantial input from the scientific community and the public.

b. The director of NIH should present the scientific rationale for trans-NIH budgeting to the relevant committees of Congress, including a proposed target for investment in trans-NIH initiatives across all institutes. For example, an average target of 5% of overall NIH funding in the first year, growing to 10% or more over 4-5 years, may be appropriate.

c. The appropriations committees should annually review budget justifications and testimony from the NIH director and from individual IC directors about the participation of each unit in the planned trans-NIH initiatives and the portion of their budgets so directed. Congress should include budget targets in the appropriations report language. The Committee recommends beginning with 5% of the overall NIH budget.

d. To ensure that each IC uses the target proportion of its budget for trans-NIH initiatives of its choosing, that proportion of the annual appropriation to each unit should be treated as "in escrow" until the NIH director affirms that the unit has committed to its expenditure for the identified trans-NIH initiatives.

e. The President should include in the budget request, and Congress should include in the NIH appropriation for OD, funds to support an appropriate number of additional full-time staff to conduct the trans-NIH planning process and "jump-start" the initiatives that emerge from this process.

To carry out the responsibilities of managing, planning, and coordinating the programs of NIH's 27 ICs, the NIH director is assisted by a number of staff units collectively called Office of the Director (OD) Operations. The budget for OD Operations has not grown in proportion to NIH's research funding and is inadequate for the effective management of the organization. When unforeseen needs surface, the OD is likely to have to "pass the hat" to the ICs to gather the additional resources needed.

Recommendation 5: *Strengthen the Office of the NIH Director*
The Office of the Director should be given a more adequate budget to support its management roles or greater discretionary authority to reprogram funding from the earmarked components of its budget when necessary to meet unanticipated needs. In particular, if the director is given the responsibility and authority to conduct NIH-wide planning for trans-NIH initiatives, the director's budget will need to be amplified to take the costs of such planning into account.

The earmarking of funds by Congress for the establishment and continuation of programmatic offices in OD sometimes limits the director's flexibility and fluidity of resources, as well as his or her ability to effect change across the organization. It is difficult to ascertain whether the programmatic offices within OD have achieved their intended goals. The time may be right to assess the effect that the programmatic offices in OD have had, including their role in the NIH director's policy and planning processes, whether the programs have clear goals, and whether there is a need to "sunset" an office once it achieves its goals. The Committee believes that the process recommended in Chapter 4 for evaluating the merits of proposed additions to or subtractions from the list of ICs should also be applied to the creation of new offices in OD itself.

Recommendation 6: *Establish a Process for Creating New OD Offices and Programs*
The public process recommended in Chapter 4 (Recommendation 2) for evaluating a proposal to create a new institute or center or to consolidate or dissolve institutes or centers should also be used for a proposal to create, consolidate, or dissolve offices in OD. The process should be used to evaluate the scientific needs, opportunities, and consequences of the proposed change, the likelihood of resources being available to support it, and public support for it.

The pressures that exist in organizational environments such as NIH's may make it difficult to undertake high-risk research—even though such research may offer potentially high payoff. The Committee also believes that there is a need for a director's Special Projects Program that is outside the budgets of the ICs and is funded as an OD line item. The goal of the program would be to provide a mechanism to augment the funding of high-risk, innovative research projects. In a broad sense, the Committee imagines the program to be patterned after the Defense Advanced Research Projects Agency (DARPA).

Recommendation 7: *Create a Director's Special Projects Program*
A discrete program, the director's Special Projects Program, should be established in OD to fund the initiation of high-risk, exceptionally innovative research projects offering high potential payoff. The program should have its own leader, who reports to the director of NIH, and a staff of short-term (2-4 years) program managers to manage identified projects with advice on program content from extramural panels. The program should be structured to permit rapid review and initiation of promising projects; if peer review is deemed appropriate, the program should use peer review panels created specifically for it and charged with selecting high-risk, high-potential return projects. Congress should be prepared to provide new funding in the amount of $100 million, growing to as much as $1 billion per year for this endeavor, and commit to support it for at least 8-10 years so that a sufficient number of projects can reach fruition and a

full assessment of program efforts can be made. A program review should be conducted during the fifth year to provide mid-course guidance.

The Committee is convinced that the Intramural Research Program (IRP) of NIH should not be merely an internal extension of the extramural community but rather should be doing distinctive research that the extramural community cannot or will not undertake. The Committee believes that too little weight has been placed on potentially distinctive contributions of the IRP and that both uniqueness and quality should be essential justifications of the IRP.

Recommendation 8: *Promote Innovation and Risk Taking in Intramural Research*
The intramural research program should consist of research and training programs that complement and are distinguished from those in the extramural community and the private sector. The intramural program's special status obligates it to take risks and be innovative. Regular in-depth review of each component of the intramural program should occur to ensure continuing excellence. Allocation of resources to the intramural program should be closely tied to accomplishments and opportunities. Inter-institute and intramural-extramural collaborations should be supported and enhanced.

ACCOUNTABILITY, ADMINISTRATION, AND LEADERSHIP

Public accountability and leadership are key aspects of NIH's stewardship of the biomedical enterprise. The Committee has suggested several ways for NIH to enhance its public accountability and ensure the continuing vitality of its leadership.

The current deficiencies in information management methods and infrastructure to collect, analyze, and report level-of-investment data in a timely fashion must be addressed. The problem requires the development of an NIH-wide agreement on what to track and publish and of a single method for coding data that uses consistent definitions and deals with the uncertainties inherent in counting research when it is only related but not directly applicable to a specific topic. Once developed, the statistics should be kept current and their accuracy ensured through quality control. NIH must also improve its tracking and analysis of the research accomplishments of scientists trained and supported with NIH funds.

Recommendation 9: *Standardize Data and Information Management Systems*
For purposes of meeting its responsibilities for effective management, accountability, and transparency, NIH must enhance its capacity for the timely collection, thoughtful analysis, and accurate reporting of the nature and status of its research and training programs and public health advances. Data should be collected consistently across institutes and centers and submitted to a centralized information management system.

The vision of the NIH leadership regarding accountability and the procedures and structures that the leadership adopts to enhance it are perhaps the most important ingredients in the complex mix of policies and strategies that enable NIH to meet its responsibilities to all its constituents. Leadership and vision may influence particularly the extent to which accountability is reinforced and implemented at diverse levels of the NIH system, from top management through staff to individual intramural and extramural investigators. In the current NIH environment, reviews of the performance of senior members of management—a form of public accountability—are too informal and ad hoc to be effective. Moreover, the processes and criteria for review are not obvious or well defined. These reviews should consider the extent to which the institute/center director promotes the effectiveness of NIH as an overall entity, including supporting trans-NIH initiatives. By communicating, as appropriate, the results of reviews to the NIH director's advisory groups, the IC directors can demonstrate an additional level of accountability. While some aspects of a review should be held as confidential, those elements that relate directly to the mission and objectives of NIH should be made available to the director's advisors.

The Committee also believes that a healthy degree of turnover in leadership is critical for sustaining the vitality of a research organization. It would provide opportunities for leading scientists across the nation to leave their positions for a set period to come to NIH as a form of public service to provide effective scientific leadership to critical elements of the nation's biomedical enterprise.

Recommendation 10: *Set Terms and Conditions for IC Director Appointments and Improve IC Director Review Process*

a. All IC directors should be appointed for 5-year terms. The possibility of a second and final term of 5 years should be based on the recommendation of the director of NIH, which should include consideration of the findings of an external review of job performance. The authority to hire and fire IC directors should be transferred from the secretary of Health and Human Services to the NIH director.

b. The director of NIH should establish a process of annual review for the performance of every IC director in terms of his or her effectiveness in fulfilling scientific and administrative responsibilities. The results of such reviews should be communicated, as appropriate, to the Advisory Committee to the director and/or the Council of Public Representatives.

The Committee concluded that review and revitalization of OD is an essential prerequisite for accountability and leadership. It noted that the National Science Foundation Act of 1950 creates a term of 6 years for the National Science Foundation director and concluded that this has been a good model for creating a system of accountability and periodic review that has the possibility of transcending changes in administrations.

Recommendation 11: *Set Terms and Conditions for the NIH Director Appointment*
The NIH director, appointed by the President, should serve for a term of 6 years unless removed sooner by the President. The possibility of a second and final term of 6 years should be based on a positive external review of performance and the recommendation of the secretary of Health and Human Services.

The committee believes that the special status granted the National Cancer Institute (NCI) by the National Cancer Act should be re-examined. Because the President appoints the NCI director and the NCI budget bypasses the NIH director, it is possible that an unnecessary rift is created between the goals, mission, and leadership of NIH and those of NCI. For scientific and administrative reasons, this special status should be reconsidered.

Recommendation 12: *Reconsider the Status of the National Cancer Institute*
Congress should reassess the provisions of the National Cancer Act of 1971, particularly as they affect the authority of the NIH director to hire senior management and plan and coordinate the NIH budget and its programs in their entirety.

Like other federal science agencies, NIH makes extensive use of advisory committees (variously known as study sections, councils, boards, etc.) of nonfederal scientists, health advocacy representatives, and others to ensure the best possible input of expertise and additional perspectives on the evaluation of programs and the development of policies and priorities. NIH had over 140 chartered advisory committees as of May 2002, more than any other federal agency. The secretary of Health and Human Services appoints 32 committees, the NIH director appoints 74, and the President appoints 2. In the appointment process, the President generally follows the recommendations of the secretary and the secretary generally follows the advice of the NIH and institute directors in filling positions, although they add their own candidates from time to time. At times in the past, administrations have tried to exert greater control over NIH, and there has been conflict over the perceived politicization of the advisory committee appointment process. The Committee believes that it is essential that members be appointed to these advisory groups because of their ability to provide scientific or public health expertise to the review and approval of awards and policies. They should not be selected to advance political or ideological positions.

There are substantial differences among institutes in the uses and roles of advisory councils; some are actively involved in establishing institute goals, and others are restricted to *pro forma* actions, with little advice or involvement sought by institute personnel. Advisory councils should routinely and consistently be consulted in the priority setting and planning processes of an institute, have active involvement in decisions regarding issuance of program announcements and requests for applications, and work to ensure that the institute is held accountable in reaching its goals and communicating with the public. The manner in which institute directors interact with their advisory councils should be a criterion for IC director reviews.

Recommendation 13: *Retain Integrity in Appointments to Advisory Councils and Reform Advisory Council Activity and Membership Criteria*

a. Appointments to advisory councils should be based solely on a person's scientific or clinical expertise or his or her commitment to and involvement in issues of relevance to the mission of the institute or center.

b. The advisory council system should be thoroughly reformed across NIH to ensure that these bodies are consistently and sufficiently independent and are routinely involved in priority-setting and planning discussions. Councils should be effectively engaged in discussions with IC leadership to enhance accountability, facilitate translation of goals and activities to the scientific community and the public, and provide feedback to the IC director. To achieve sufficient independence and avoid conflicts of interest, a substantial proportion of a council's scientific membership should consist of persons whose primary source of research support is derived from a different institute or center or from outside NIH.

Although it is desirable to keep administrative and overhead costs as low as possible, appropriate funding for these costs is essential to the effectiveness of any organization, including those that sponsor research and training programs. At NIH, the resources for those functions (for example, management of extramural activities, some intramural research program costs, program development, priority setting, education and outreach, acquisition and maintenance of new information technology systems, professional development, and facilities management) flow through the Research Management and Support (RMS) budgets of the various units that make up NIH. In the early 1990s, Congress imposed limitations on RMS that restricted its growth. In the middle 1990s, RMS was reduced, and little growth has been allowed since. In FY 2001, RMS represented 3.3% of the total NIH budget, down from 4.5% in 1995. The RMS share of the total NIH budget has decreased every year since FY 1993. The committee feels that the effectiveness of NIH is now imperiled by the lack of adequate resources to provide appropriate support both for its primary research mission and for meeting its accountability responsibilities.

Recommendation 14: *Increase Funding for Research Management and Support*
Congress should increase the appropriation for RMS to reflect more accurately the essential administrative costs required to effectively operate a world class $27 billion/year research organization effectively. Moreover, when additional

congressional mandates are imposed on NIH through the appropriations process, they should include funds to cover necessary administrative costs.

Whether needs and opportunities will be accommodated in existing NIH units or proliferation or consolidation will occur in the near future is an issue to be addressed by future administrations, Congress, the scientific community, and the public. NIH will continue to be shaped by the dynamics of many interacting constituencies and influences. Interests will converge or conflict, depending on the issue. The degree of convergence and divergence will continue to be influenced by other important factors such as the level of annual congressional appropriations to NIH. The recommendations made in this report are intended to help NIH to continue to be responsive, accountable, and effective in its leading role in the vast international humanitarian enterprise of biomedical research aimed at a better understanding of the human condition, the prevention and relief of disease, and the promotion of good health throughout the stages of life.

Summary of Recommendations

1. Assure that centralization of management functions will not undermine NIH's ability to identify, fund, and manage the best research and training.
2. Create a public process for considering proposed changes in the number of NIH institutes or centers.
3. Strengthen the overall NIH clinical research effort through consolidation of programs and creation of a new leadership position.
4. Enhance and increase trans-NIH strategic planning and funding.
5. Strengthen the office of the NIH director.
6. Establish a process for creating new OD offices and programs.
7. Create a Director's Special Projects Program to support high-risk, high-potential payoff research.
8. Promote innovation and risk-taking in intramural research.
9. Standardize level-of-investment data and information management systems.
10. Set terms and conditions for IC director appointments and improve the IC director review process.
11. Set terms and conditions for the NIH director appointment.
12. Reconsider the special status of the National Cancer Institute.
13. Retain integrity in appointments to advisory councils and reform advisory council activity and membership criteria.
14. Increase funding for Research Management and Support.

1

Introduction

By any measure, the National Institutes of Health (NIH) is an important component of a vast international humanitarian enterprise aimed at a better understanding of human health, prevention and relief of the burdens of disease, and promotion of good health throughout the stages of life. It is an optimistic endeavor predicated on the belief that human life can be improved through scientific investigations coupled with the rational and ethical applications of their findings. It is an enterprise full of moral relevance because it contributes to the interests of current and future generations and to the commitment to reduce health disparities.

In *Democracy in America* (1835), French statesman Alexis de Tocqueville wrote of what he perceived as the peculiarly American pursuit of good health. Although achieving that goal remains elusive for many Americans, since the middle 1900s the US government has invested generously in biomedical research,[1] believing that such activities would have great long-term benefits for the health of American citizens and others. There is broad agreement among the American people, Congress, and the Executive Branch that investing in biomedical research is socially desirable because of its health benefits, its capacity to increase understanding of the human condition, and its potential to directly or indirectly yield economic dividends. The assumption that federally funded scientific research generates economic and other benefits for the country has been fundamental to US science policy since the end of

---

[1] Biomedical research in this report includes all the following categories of research: fundamental (basic), applied, behavioral, bioengineering and biotechnology, clinical, dental, health, health services, nursing, outcomes, population-based, prevention, public health, rehabilitative, and therapeutic.

World War II (Bush, 1945). As Donald Stokes pointed out in *Pasteur's Quadrant* (1997), the American public deeply values such investment in science "not only for what it is, but what it's for."

The investment in human health improvement has paid handsome dividends. Age-adjusted rates of heart disease and stroke continue to decline, there has been a modest but encouraging decrease in cancer death rates, life expectancy continues to rise, infant mortality rates are falling, and the field of genomics has advanced to the point where promising new therapeutic agents are under development by biotechnology and pharmaceutical companies. The knowledge gained from biomedical research and the large cohorts of highly trained biomedical scientists continue to be among the nation's most valuable resources. Nevertheless, new public health concerns, chronic illnesses, emerging or re-emerging infectious diseases, and persistent health disparities constitute continuing challenges for our biomedical and health care research enterprise.

For nearly 65 years, the federal agency primarily responsible for sponsoring and conducting biomedical research has been the NIH. NIH is one of eight agencies of the Public Health Service (PHS), which is part of the Department of Health and Human Services (DHHS).[2] NIH accounts for about 80% of federal funding of biomedical research and development (R&D); the Department of Defense (DOD) is the second largest supporter, at 6% (NIH, 2002). Since its formation, Congress and the Executive Branch have supported steady increases in NIH's budget. NIH is the largest public source of funding for biomedical research in the world, with an annual budget of about $27 billion. In early 2003, Congress approved an FY 2003 budget containing a 16% increase over the previous year that completed the planned 5-year doubling of NIH's budget.

NIH, by most accounts, has long been considered one of the most effective and well-managed elements of the federal government and a centerpiece of its R&D system. From one categorical institute at the end of World War II, it has evolved into a federation of 27 major institutes and centers as of 2003 (see Chapter 2 for further discussion), each conducting and sponsoring research and related activities on aspects of human health and disease through grants and contracts to scientists in universities and other nonfederal research institutions.

To ensure its continued effectiveness, NIH must respond in a rapidly changing environment that is characterized by a renewed appreciation of the complexity of human biology; the increasing need for cooperation among biomedical and related disciplines and scientists working in different sectors; growing investments in biomedical research by the US corporate sector and other countries; the need to deal

---

[2]The other seven are the Agency for Healthcare Research and Quality, the Agency for Toxic Substances and Disease Registry, the Centers for Disease Control and Prevention, the Food and Drug Administration, the Health Resources and Services Administration, the Indian Health Service, and the Substance Abuse and Mental Health Services Administration.

with new institutional arrangements in the broader scientific enterprise that generate additional incentives, conflicts, and constraints; and developments on the scientific frontier that, for example, require changes in the technologies used, the organization of research teams, and the active engagement of participants in clinical research. Equally important are the effective management of the rapidly expanded NIH budget and the challenge of managing the many organizational components of NIH—institutes, centers, and offices.

ONE IMPETUS FOR THIS REPORT

A persistent subject in discussions about the organization and future of NIH is the continued growth in the number of institutes, centers, and other programmatic and organizational components that have been mandated by congressional initiative in response to the demands of various interest groups. Several NIH directors have raised concerns about such growth. Former Director James Wyngaarden, in congressional testimony arguing against the creation of another institute in 1982, pointed out that "there is virtually no end to the possibilities for creation of additional categorical institutes." From a scientific viewpoint, Wyngaarden noted the mismatch between the categorical structure of NIH and trends in research toward investigating the basic life processes that underlie all health and disease and away from the symptoms of specific diseases in isolation. From a managerial point of view, Wyngaarden raised the question of whether organizational complexity tends to be counterproductive (U.S. Congress, 1981).

Harold Varmus, the most recent NIH director to suggest that the agency is becoming unmanageable through continued proliferation, opposed the establishment of NIH's two newest units, the National Institute of Biomedical Imaging and Bioengineering (NIBIB) and the Center for Minority Health and Health Disparities (NCMHD). He argued that establishing program coordination units in the director's office was preferable to creating new institutes and centers for cross-cutting fields (such as bioimaging) that should not be isolated as separate entities. He also expressed a disinclination to add to the number of units that have to be managed.[3]

Although he began to raise the issue in various forums during the last years of his tenure as NIH director (Dennis, 1999), Varmus laid out his analysis and proposed solution most fully in an article published in *Science* (Varmus, 2001) after his departure from NIH. He acknowledged the political advantages of establishing new institutes and centers but argued that NIH would be more effective scientifically and more manageable if it were organized into a far smaller number of larger institutes

---

[3]For example, Congress recommended that NIH establish an office of Bioimaging and Bioengineering, an idea that former NIH Director Harold Varmus welcomed. However, Varmus cautioned that establishing a new Institute of Bioengineering and Bioimaging was not a good idea because such activities benefit more by being distributed among the full range of institutes and centers at NIH (NIH, 1999).

organized around broad fields of science.[4] Consolidating the existing institutes into five entities "would organize the science in a rational way" (Dennis, 1999).

Others, including many biomedical investigators, argue that at the current time the elimination of institutes, centers, or offices that focus on particular sets of problems would mean that research on the problems would not receive sufficient attention and funding and that a consolidation of units would reduce congressional and public support. Those arguments were put forth by many of the organizations and individuals that wrote or spoke to the committee. Moreover, there is a perception that given the substantial increases in resources and the vast expansion of the biomedical enterprise, the addition of institutes and centers has provided for the expression of a broader set of priorities and expanded political support and budget success both for the specific interests involved and for NIH in the aggregate. While everyone understands that this expansion cannot and should not continue indefinitely, many see no particular difficulty with the current number of institutes and centers.

Many of the arguments against the formation of additional institutes and centers have focused on the adverse managerial and programmatic consequences at the NIH level (the opposite of the arguments for new institutes that stress the beneficial consequences of having one institute focused on a disease category or set of related problems)—the likelihood that a new institute or center will increase the share of the budget going to overhead because each institute has a director, senior staff, and administrative units, although some of these would be needed even if the program were kept or established in an existing unit.

Other arguments against adding institutes have had substantive grounds. In particular, there has been recurrent concern that adding an institute in a particular field could dilute, rather than concentrate, efforts in it. For example, many were concerned that the new NIBIB would reduce the commitment of other institutes to important opportunities in biomedical imaging and bioengineering. The same argument was made against creating the separate NCMHD: there was concern that establishing such a center would lead other institutes and centers to decrease their commitments to work in minority health.

---

[4]In 2001, Varmus proposed a redistribution of NIH into six units of approximately equal sizes and budgets. Five of these would be categorical institutes, committed mainly to groups of diseases: the National Cancer Institute, the National Brain Institute, the National Institute for Internal Medicine Research, the National Institute for Human Development, and the National Institute for Microbial and Environmental Medicine. Each of these would contain several major divisions for extramural research and an intramural research program. Each would also house offices to coordinate research training, international science, minority and women's health, and other activities, both within and among the five institutes. The sixth unit, NIH Central, would be led by the NIH director, to whom the directors of the five institutes would report. NIH Central would have responsibility for policies across NIH (e.g., on intellectual property, personnel management, or training programs), the peer-review process, scientific infrastructure (e.g., information technology, buildings and facilities, including the intramural Clinical Research Center), and thematic coordination (through links to the offices in each of the five institutes).

All institutes and most centers are legislatively mandated, receive their own funding, and enjoy a constituency base that, given other characteristics of NIH's environment, can reduce the organizational flexibility that less federated organizational structures give industry and many other government agencies, such as the National Science Foundation (NSF). In addition, as the number of institute and center directorships has increased, the recruiting and administrative burden on the NIH director has become substantial. Although some argue that NIH is becoming unmanageable, others believe that this is not the case and that substantial consolidation might not be programmatically desirable or politically feasible. In fact, some believe that the complex decentralized organization developed over the years has made NIH *more* effective in responding to research opportunities and public needs and aspirations and is an important source of its success (Congressional Budget Office, 2002).

In addition to the issues surrounding the proliferation of units, recent changes in biomedical science and how it is conducted may also raise questions beyond the narrow matter of the number of components in the organization. For example, research is becoming more interdisciplinary, more dependent on a common set of research tools and technologies (including costly large-scale infrastructure, such as supercomputers and imaging machines), and more focused on fundamental processes that underlie many diseases.[5] Many of those developments increase the benefits of a strategic and coordinated effort among institutes and centers in some fields and may call for a more strategic NIH-wide approach to emerging challenges than has been traditional at NIH. Those emerging opportunities do not necessarily argue for a reduction in the number of units at NIH so much as for a change in the qualitative nature of the work conducted and the depth and breadth of interactions among the units.

Other trends also have caused some to believe that a review of the organizational structure of the agency is necessary. For example, demographics and patterns of illness in society are changing and investment by the private sector is growing, which has altered the terrain of some areas of research in a manner that could call for an adjustment in the role of NIH within the broader biomedical enterprise. Pharmaceutical and biotechnology companies now spend more than NIH on research and development—well over $46 billion per year (Pharmaceutical Research and Manufacturers of America, 2001; Biotechnology Industry Organization, 2003). In addition, the Bayh-Dole Act (PL 96-517, Patent and Trademark Act Amendments of 1980) created a uniform patent policy among the many federal agencies that fund research, enabling small businesses and nonprofit organizations, including universities, to retain title to inventions made in federally funded research programs, thereby creating a new congressionally mandated responsibility of NIH to

---

[5]These trends have been cited by NIH leaders. See, for example, the remarks of Director Elias Zerhouni at a field hearing held by a subcommittee of the House Science Committee (Jenkins, 2002a) and presentations by Acting Director Ruth Kirschstein (Kirschstein, 2001; Haley, 2001).

further technology transfer and commercialization of its research results by the private sector.

As a result of the steady stream of change, there have been persistent and growing concerns in Congress and in some parts of the scientific community about whether NIH has become too fragmented to address effectively the most important biomedical and health challenges or to respond quickly enough to health emergencies or economic challenges. Despite those persistent concerns, NIH has never been administratively reorganized in any substantial way, but only added to, despite vast changes in the landscape of science and the nation's health concerns during the last half century.

CONGRESSIONAL REQUEST AND STATEMENT OF TASK

In report language that accompanied the FY 2001 appropriation act, Congress directed NIH to have the National Academy of Sciences study "whether the current structure and organization of NIH are optimally configured for the scientific needs of the twenty-first century."[6] Senate report 106-293 states:

> The Committee is extremely pleased with the scientific advances that have been made over the past several years due to the Nation's support for biomedical research at NIH. However, the Committee also notes the proliferation of new entities at NIH, raising concerns about coordination. While the Committee continues to have confidence in NIH's ability to fund outstanding research and to ensure that new knowledge will benefit all Americans, the fundamental changes in science that have occurred lead us to question whether the current NIH structure and organization are optimally configured for the scientific needs of the Twenty-first Century. Therefore, the Committee has provided to the NIH Director sufficient funds to undertake, through the National Academy of Sciences, a study of the structure of NIH.

In response to the congressional request, the goal of this study was to determine the optimal NIH organizational structure, given the context of 21st century biomedical science. The following specific questions were to be addressed:

1. Are there general principles by which NIH should be organized?
2. Does the current structure reflect these principles, or should NIH be restructured?
3. If restructuring is recommended, what should the new structure be?

---

[6]HRpt 106-1033, "Conference Report to Accompany H.R. 4577 - Making Omnibus Consolidated and Emergency Supplemental Appropriations for Fiscal Year 2001," December 15, 2000, endorsed the language in the Senate report calling for the NAS study of the NIH structure and asked for a report within a year of the appointment of the new NIH Director. See SRpt 106-293, "Departments of Labor, Health and Human Services, and Education and Related Agencies Appropriation Bill, 2001," May 12, 2000.

4. How will the proposed new structure improve NIH's ability to conduct biomedical research and training, and accommodate organizational growth in the future?
5. How would the proposed new structure overcome current weaknesses, and what new problems might it introduce?

The Committee on the Organizational Structure of the National Institutes of Health was formed to ensure that the views of the basic science, clinical medicine, and health advocacy communities were all adequately represented. The Committee also included persons who were experienced in the management of large and complex organizations, including a former NIH director, two former NIH institute directors, a former university president, two individuals with backgrounds as senior managers of major industrial entities, and a specialist in organizational issues. Several Committee members also had considerable experience in government operations.

The Committee held six 2-day meetings over the 10 months between July 2002 and April 2003. In its initial meetings it invited past and present representatives of Congress, NIH, voluntary health groups, scientific and professional societies, and industry to provide perspectives on the issues before them (see Appendix A). In addition, the Committee met publicly with the current NIH director as well as several former directors. Committee members and staff also heard presentations from or interviewed NIH staff in the offices of policy and planning, budget, finance, and intramural research, and met with directors of 18 institutes or centers. Data about NIH programs and budgets were requested from NIH staff as the need emerged. Prior reports conducted about and for NIH were reviewed, as was the relevant literature. In addition, the Committee commissioned a background paper tracing the history and evolution of NIH and its institutes as a starting point for its deliberations (McGeary and Smith, 2002). Finally, several Committee members conducted town meetings at their home institutions and elsewhere, inviting scientists, administrators, and students to contribute their perspectives. Thus, the Committee was able to hear, consider, and discuss a diverse range of facts and opinions about the organizational structure of NIH. Its final report and recommendations are, however, based on the Committee's assessment of both the information available and current trends in biomedical science and health.

THE COMMITTEE'S RESPONSE TO ITS CHARGE

This study focused on the organizational structure of NIH, but that cannot be addressed satisfactorily without considering the mission of NIH, some of its key processes, and the scientific and social-political environment in which NIH activities take place. Although a long series of past reviews of NIH helped inform committee deliberations, the nature of the charge and the 1-year period allowed for deliberations constrained the development, character, and scope of the recommendations that the Committee could credibly put forward. Most important, the committee was not asked to address NIH's research priorities or the quality and effectiveness of the wide array of research and advanced training programs that NIH undertakes or sponsors.

Even a relatively narrowly defined focus on the organizational structure of NIH was challenging because of the need to disentangle structure, procedure, policies, achievements, criticisms, and priorities. For example, the Committee debated whether its charge referred solely to the number of institutes and centers that can be effectively and responsibly managed or could it also assess the role and authority of the NIH director? Should the nature, role, and scope of the intramural research program be discussed because the program is a key structural element of NIH? Over the years many talented and energetic scientists have occupied various leadership positions at NIH and introduced a wide variety of innovative organizational initiatives. Many of these initiatives have been successfully implemented in individual institutes, centers, and offices, but they have not moved easily from unit to unit or survived changes in leadership. What managerial mechanisms might ensure the widespread adoption of best practices by the institutes, and how might they be adopted or strengthened in place of or in conjunction with structural reorganization? One could pose numerous additional questions in an attempt to understand and define the set of activities, processes, and procedures encompassed by the term "organizational structure." And such questions cannot even be approached without considering the role and mission of NIH.

The Committee's view of those complexities was governed by the desire to be of some practical assistance to all those who wish NIH to continue to be an effective—indeed, outstanding—organization. The Committee therefore took its task to include assessing the organizational configuration of NIH—both its quantitative and qualitative aspects—and the key processes and authorities that play roles in NIH-wide decision-making. Although the borders between structure, mission, and priorities are themselves not well defined, the Committee tried not to take too expansive a view of its responsibilities. In addition, Elias Zerhouni, the current NIH director, suggested to the committee at its first meeting that it would be useful for the committee to concentrate on and assess eight specific issues:

1. The effectiveness of governance mechanisms.
2. The effectiveness of decision-making processes across and within the institutes.
3. The balance between centralization and decentralization.
4. The need for better management tools (NIH-wide standards and methods).
5. The development of mechanisms to allocate (or redirect) resources across NIH.
6. Mechanisms for coordination of science.
7. The ability of the NIH leadership to hold institutes accountable.
8. The need for strategic human resources policies.

Based on the advice it received from former and current NIH directors as well as its conversations with congressional staff, throughout its deliberations the Committee kept a number of broadly conceived organizational ideas in mind. First, scholars of organizational management (e.g., Waterman et al., 1980) have long recognized that there is more to "organization" than structure. An organization's ability to make effective changes is influenced by a multiplicity of factors beyond the number of units on or shape of its organizational chart, for example strategy, structure, systems, staff capabilities, shared values, and behavior. "Systems" refers to all the formal and informal processes and procedures that organizations rely on to function. The word "organized" calls the question: Organized to do what? The answer typically is: Organized to build new institutional capability or new skill—in this case, for example, the institutional skill to adapt research and training programs to the new demands of science. To respond to change, an organization must work out its *strategy*—preferably mixed strategies—and, if necessary, *restructure* in order to implement those strategies. Also it will have to change other dimensions of the way it organizes itself to respond. In line with these views, the Committee believes that many potential changes in aspects of NIH other than the number of blocks on its organizational chart could improve its overall effectiveness and help it to stay at the cutting edge of biomedical research.

Therefore the Committee considered numerous proposals for restructuring NIH in great detail[7] but did not focus exclusively on whether or not there should be a widespread consolidation of NIH's institutes and centers. Rather, it took a more general approach, namely to inquire if there were any significant organizational changes—including the widespread consolidation of institutes and centers—that would allow NIH to be even more successful in the future. Although the Committee discussed on numerous occasions the advisability of the widespread consolidation of NIH, it eventually came to believe that this was not the best path for NIH to take at this time.

It is important to understand that the structure of any large and complex organization, such as NIH, is not the tidy result of a compact set of compelling

---

[7]In their background paper prepared for this Committee, McGeary and Smith (2002) summarized the published responses to the Varmus proposal and the results of their interviews on this topic. In addition, at its inaugural meeting, July 30-31, 2002, the Committee heard from Bernadine Healy, NIH director from 1991 to 1993, who suggested grouping NIH in four quite different "clusters": 1) federal laboratories and the clinical center to deal with emergency issues; 2) health and disease institutes; 3) medical and scientific institutes; and 4) a national research capacity (e.g., NCRR, NLM, large clinical trials capability). Dr. Healy was not opposed to forming more institutes—she even suggested two new units for nutrition and rehabilitation. She noted, however, that abolishing institutes is easier said than done. This was reiterated by former Illinois Representative and House Appropriations Subcommittee Chair John Porter, who told the group that any attempt to eliminate individual institutes will likely meet strong political resistance. He urged the committee to think of ways to eliminate duplication and increase consolidation and accountability.

propositions emanating from organizational theory any more than the particular organization of our complex pluralistic democracy is the result solely of the inspired thinking of political philosophers. The latter is instead the outcome of our particular form of politics and, therefore, heavily influenced by our particular history and evolving cultural commitments. It is very much the same way with NIH. It would be naïve to assume that NIH was or should be organized exclusively along the lines dictated either by the imperatives of the scientific agenda or the priorities of any other single set of interests with a concern about promoting health-related research and advanced biomedical training. Rather NIH's existing structure is the result of a set of complex evolving social and political negotiations among a variety of constituencies including the Congress, the administration, the scientific community, the health advocacy community, and others interested in research, research training, and public policy related to health. Indeed the history of NIH provides clear evidence that each of these communities has always had a variety of views on the appropriate organization of NIH. From any particular point of view or for any particular set of interests, the current situation is not only imperfect, but is certainly not one that either the Congress or the scientific community would designate *ab initio*. Rather it has evolved as a very useful and largely productive outcome of a series of political and social negotiations that took place over time. This outcome is typical of the design of important social organizations in a pluralistic democracy. NIH has become an organization that balances its many interests and the Committee felt that any major modification at this point in time should focus directly on enhancing NIH's capacity to pursue major, but time-limited, strategic objectives that cut across all the institutes and to acquire a special ability to pursue more high-risk, high-return projects. It was our view that at this moment the widespread consolidation of institutes and centers should not be a high priority as the benefits to be gained would not sufficiently offset the costs involved, particularly when there are other available options that could achieve the same benefits.

What does the Committee mean by "costs"? At a minimum, because Congress created the institutes, dissolving or merging institutes would require congressional action. Any thoughtful major reorganization would necessitate a lengthy and complex information gathering and decision making process that would include numerous congressional hearings involving members of Congress, congressional staff, and a wide variety of interests in the various health advocacy and scientific communities. Our discussions, correspondence, and meetings made it quite clear that there would be very little agreement among these communities on what the right way to reorganize NIH is, and there would probably be dozens of conflicting ideas in play and few clear avenues for narrowing these down. Moreover these discussions and negotiations would be long and contentious ones and with a quite uncertain outcome. More importantly, the Committee is firmly convinced that many of the goals that might be achieved through large-scale consolidation of institutes could also be achieved more rapidly and effectively through other organizational and administrative mechanisms, as recommended in this report.

Nevertheless, the Committee did feel that no organization as important as NIH should remain frozen in organization space and that some regular, thoughtful, and publicly transparent mechanism is required to allow changes to take place at appropriate times. Although the Committee does believe that the consolidation of two pairs of institutes is appropriate at this time, it felt that this issue ought to have the benefit of the public process it has recommended.

Thus, as laid out in this report, the Committee did not find a compelling intellectual argument for widespread consolidation of institutes and centers at this time. It did, however, identify numerous opportunities for organizational change to improve the agency's responsiveness and flexibility and makes several suggestions for adopting an array of strategies to better accomplish NIH's research mission.

The Committee was aware that all organizational changes, however well thought out, carry both potential risks and benefits, and it has done its best to sort these out. It also recognized that the decentralized structure of NIH, which allows many people throughout the scientific and advocacy communities to help to set priorities, has been and should continue to be an integral element in NIH's success. The current structure of NIH allows the public to see its many faces. The Committee believes that this has been a very useful organizational response to a complicated set of scientific and political influences. The Committee was particularly mindful of the need to sustain the coalition that has made NIH the success that it is today. In addition, the Committee kept the enormous benefits of investigator-initiated grants, including those focused on fundamental research, firmly in mind during its deliberations. Finally, the Committee understood that the quality of leadership and decision-making at all levels, as opposed to administrative structures, is central to NIH's ongoing vitality. In the long run, the recruitment of outstanding leadership, the commitment to individual scientists as the main sources of new discoveries, and reliance on the competitive review system for determining awards will continue to be essential to NIH's continuing success.

That NIH has been working well does not mean that it could not work better if—in response to changes on the scientific frontier, to changes in health concerns, or to other important environmental shifts—some organizational changes were made. The intent of this report is to assess the current organizational structure of NIH and to suggest modifications that might be appropriate to make NIH even more effective in supporting research essential to the long-term goal of improving human health.

GENERAL PRINCIPLES BY WHICH NIH SHOULD BE ORGANIZED

NIH accomplishes its objectives through the design, organization, administration, and management of extramural and intramural research and training programs and the provision of specialized research facilities that support the programs. In broad scope, NIH's priorities focus on scientific research that is most likely to shape the understanding, diagnosis, treatment, and prevention of society's most important health challenges. That focus includes strong support of fundamental scientific research that is aimed at improving our understanding of organisms, processes, biological systems, and individual and societal risk factors broadly believed to be relevant to human health. It also embraces support of graduate and postgraduate training needed to ensure an adequate supply of scientists to continue to study those important health concerns.

An evaluation of NIH's priorities requires explicit recognition of a number of interrelated factors. Most important in this respect is an understanding of the evolving nature of the scientific enterprise, which includes not only the changing nature of science itself, but also the evolving role of other institutions and disciplines, both here and abroad, that have generally similar aims as well as the changing nature of our health concerns. Recognition of the global nature of medical and health problems and their relevance to the interests and health of the people of the United States warrants special mention. Finally, and perhaps most obvious, the level of resources available to NIH clearly will affect the profile and extent of NIH's activities. Effective management of its resources is especially challenging now because of the pace of scientific developments, new health priorities, the changing institutional structure of the biomedical research enterprise, and recent rapid budget growth.

In going about its task, the Committee first addressed the opening question in its statement of task: "Are there general principles by which NIH should be organized?" Only by arriving at an early determination of NIH's principal overall function and the mechanisms in place to achieve its mission could the Committee adequately address the other items in its charge. Thus, an overarching mission and the mechanisms needed to meet it became the basis of the remainder of the committee's tasks. The recommendations developed by the Committee focus on modifications in basic policies and organizational structure that are designed to assist NIH in performing its primary function.

The success of NIH in meeting its various challenges and, in particular, fulfilling its mission to improve health through the use of science to develop new knowledge has been outstanding. All those who have contributed to the creation and dynamic evolution of the NIH—the institutions it has supported, the scientists and health professionals who have created so much knowledge and understanding, and the American people and their elected representatives—have helped to reduce humankind's burden of disease, disability, and premature death. NIH has also been successful in catalyzing changes at the frontiers of science. Those changes and the recent doubling of NIH's budget make this an appropriate time to consider whether the organizational structures that have served NIH and the world so well in the past remain appropriate for its future roles.

The charge to this Committee is worded in the form of a series of questions about whether there are general principles around which NIH should be organized. In the context of evaluating NIH's organizational structure, the Committee decided to describe the principles as they relate to NIH's overall mission and the basic policies, structural and otherwise, adopted to achieve it. In the end, the Committee agreed that articulating its view of the mission of NIH would provide the appropriate foundation to guide its deliberations:

> NIH's principal mission is to serve as a mechanism for efficiently and effectively deploying federal resources across a wide array of institutions and individuals in the nation's scientific community to advance the scientific frontier and ensure research and training in fields of special relevance to human health needs.[8]

Some might view this mission as stopping short of the goals of public health, that is, not including the goal to directly improve human health. The Committee was cognizant of the tension that exists among the scientific, medical, patient, and political communities about expectations of NIH. It concluded, however, that improving health—as much as it is critically dependent on accurate and adequate science—is a goal that also involves health providers, industry, and policy makers and is influenced by social and economic factors that range far from the research mission of NIH. Moreover, NIH is but one of eight DHHS agencies charged with a health-related mission. The other agencies—Agency for Healthcare Research and Quality, the Centers for Disease Control and Prevention, the Agency for Toxic Substances and Disease Registry, the Food and Drug Administration, the Health Resources and Services Administration, the Indian Health Service, and the Substance Abuse and Mental Health Services Administration—also focus on health and complement the research mission of NIH. There is no question that these agencies must work together even more effectively to ensure that there is a continuum of federal effort and concern regarding improved health for all Americans.

Based on its view of NIH's mission, the Committee agreed that there follows from this fundamental charge a list of subprinciples or basic policies and approaches that, if adhered to, would allow NIH to achieve its mission:

1. The NIH research and training portfolio should be broad and integrated, ranging from basic to applied and from laboratory to population-based, in support of understanding health and how to improve it for all populations. The portfolio should reflect a balance between work in existing highly productive domains or disciplines and high-risk, groundbreaking, potentially paradigm-shifting work. It should be especially responsive whenever scientific opportunity and public health and health care needs overlap.
2. NIH should support research that cuts across multiple health domains and disease categories. This might require special efforts to integrate research across NIH components.
3. The NIH research and training portfolio should make special efforts to address health problems that typically do not attract substantial private

---

[8]NIH states its mission as "science in pursuit of fundamental knowledge about the nature and behavior of living systems and the application of that knowledge to extend healthy life and reduce the burdens of illness and disability" (NIH, 2001).

sector support, such as prevention, some therapeutic strategies, and many rare diseases.
4. The standards, procedures, and processes by which research and training funds are allocated should be transparent to applicants, Congress, voluntary health organizations, and the general public. Moreover, a wide variety of constituencies should have input into the setting of broad priorities.
5. Extramural research should remain the primary vehicle for carrying out NIH's mission. Open competitive peer review should be the usual mechanism guiding extramural funding decisions.
6. The intramural research program is a unique federal resource that offers an important opportunity to enhance NIH's capability to fulfill its mission. It should seek to fill distinctive roles in the nation's scientific enterprise with appropriate mechanisms of accountability and quality control.
7. As a world-class science institution, NIH should have state-of-the-art management and planning strategies and tools. A key need is the capability for retrieving comprehensive and interpretable NIH-wide data related to its various objectives.
8. There should be appropriate mechanisms to ensure the continuing review, evaluation, and appointment of senior scientific and administrative leaders at all levels of NIH.
9. Proposals for the creation, merger, or closure of institutes, centers, and offices should be considered through a process of thoughtful public deliberation that addresses potential costs, benefits, and alternatives.

ORGANIZATION OF THE REPORT

To place the Committee's analysis and recommendations in context, Chapter 2 provides background information about the evolution of the structure and organization of NIH. Chapter 3 focuses on examples of how new discoveries are changing the conduct, review, and evaluation of science and addresses whether the NIH structure is suitably configured to adapt to these changes and to promote them.

In Chapter 4, the Committee focuses on the NIH structure itself and processes for merging, consolidating, or expanding the number of its components, including a proposal to revitalize and integrate clinical research.

Chapter 5 provides ideas and suggestions for reorganization that could facilitate the conduct of increasingly important trans-NIH scientific research and enhance NIH's ability to maintain itself at the leading edge of scientific progress. The chapter proposes changes that would enhance the NIH director's authority, particularly as related to trans-NIH initiatives that should begin to constitute a larger proportion of NIH activities, mechanisms for fostering high-risk research, and the intramural research program.

Chapter 6 discusses issues related to NIH's need to be publicly and financially accountable through its advisory and review processes, data systems, leadership, and administrative efficiency, including the budgetary and administrative issues related to managing a large research organization.

Chapter 7 summarizes the recommendations made in the report in the context of their consistency with the principles and basic policies elucidated in this introduction.

SUMMARY

NIH will continue to be influenced both by scientific developments and by a changing political landscape and growth in the numbers and sophistication of scientific and health advocacy groups. Interests will converge or conflict depending on the degree to which issues are influenced by such factors as the state of the economy and the federal budget. It may seem easier to innovate and cooperate when the budget is increasing, but rapidly increasing budgets can also overwhelm good planning and long-term strategic thinking. In any case, it is clear that when budget growth slows, especially in an era of great opportunity and need, difficult decisions arise and priorities are affected.

Independently of budget issues, NIH is increasingly called on to perform in a coordinated way to address key research subjects that involve multiple institutes and to respond to immediate public health needs. An important question is whether NIH's federated and decentralized structure, as currently configured, can respond adequately and in a timely manner to those challenges. This report makes a series of recommendations aimed at increasing and enhancing NIH's ability to accomplish its mission.

2

The Evolution of NIH's Organizational Structure

The National Institutes of Health (NIH) began as a modest set of federal research laboratories supporting the public health mission of the Public Health Service. As a result of the nation's steady determination to increase its commitment to research in the biomedical and related sciences, NIH has evolved into a large and complex decentralized organization that sponsors research throughout the United States and at some sites abroad. NIH now consists of 20 institutes (including the National Library of Medicine, NLM), 7 centers, and 4 programmatic offices in the Office of the Director (OD) that are intended to coordinate activities in specific fields across NIH (Figure 2.1). Only institutes and some centers have authority to award research grants; the Clinical Center, Center for Information Technology, and Center on Scientific Review do not award research grants. The 20 institutes and 4 of the 7 centers have their own appropriations.[1] More than 40 unit heads report directly to the NIH director: the directors of the 27 institutes and centers, 12 staff offices, and four program offices.

The size and expanse of the agency are impressive. In FY 2002, NIH's budget funded 43,600 research grants and 1,600 contracts in universities, medical schools, and other research and training institutions in the United States and abroad and supported 16,700 full-time training positions.[2] NIH employs about 17,700 full-

---

[1] In addition, there are appropriations for the Office of the Director and for Buildings and Facilities, for a total of 26 separate appropriations for NIH in the Labor/Health and Human Services Appropriations Act.

[2] These figures are based on the President's budget request for FY 2003 to the Labor/Health and Human Services/Education Appropriations committees. NIH also receives some funding under the

time personnel. The intramural research program consists of more than 2,000 research projects conducted by more than 9,000 government scientists and technical support staff. The agency occupies 75 buildings on more than 300 acres in Bethesda, MD, including laboratories and a 267-bed clinical research facility. One of the institutes, the National Institute of Environmental Health Sciences (NIEHS), is in North Carolina. Additional facilities are in Baltimore, Frederick, and Poolesville, MD; Hamilton, MT; and other locations. NIH supports about 50,000 researchers at 2,000 universities and colleges, health professional schools (medicine, dental, public health, pharmacy, and nursing), teaching hospitals, independent nonprofit research institutes, and industrial laboratories in all 50 states and some other countries.

There have been unsuccessful efforts to bring other health research agencies under the NIH umbrella. For example, the National Institute for Occupational Safety and Health and the National Center for Health Services Research (now the Agency for Healthcare Research and Quality) have, at times, been considered good candidates for integration into NIH, but they were perceived as too far removed from the biomedical research mission of NIH.

INSTITUTES

The institutes are highly varied and reflect not only their particular foci and budgets but also the varied circumstances of their creation, how long they have been in existence, the nature of the scientific opportunities available, the strength of support by their advocates, and the priorities of the administration and of Congress. They are broadly similar to each other in their relationships with the NIH director, Congress, and the other institutes and centers.

The NIH institutes can be thought of as being in five general categories, although there is no optimal taxonomy for this purpose. Some are organized by disease (for example, cancer; mental health; diabetes and digestive and kidney disorders; arthritis and musculoskeletal and skin disorders; neurological diseases; allergies and infectious diseases; deafness and other communication disorders; and drug and alcohol abuse). Some are organized by organ system (for example, heart, lung and blood; and eye); some by life stage (child and human development and aging); some by field of science (for example, general medical sciences, environmental health sciences, and the human genome); and some by profession or technology (nursing, dental, biomedical imaging and bioengineering) (Morris, 1984).[3] Those institutes organized

---

Department of Veterans Affairs and Housing and Urban Development appropriation ($76 million is requested for environmental research in FY 2003) and the Balanced Budget Act of 1997 ($97 million for type 1 diabetes research is requested in FY 2003). See on-line table at http://www4.od.nih.gov/officeofbudget/CJ2003/Mechanism%20-%20Total%20Proposed%20Law.PDF.

[3]The categories and assignments through 1984 follow Morris, 1984:67. The last category, for nursing, dentistry, and imaging, has been added.

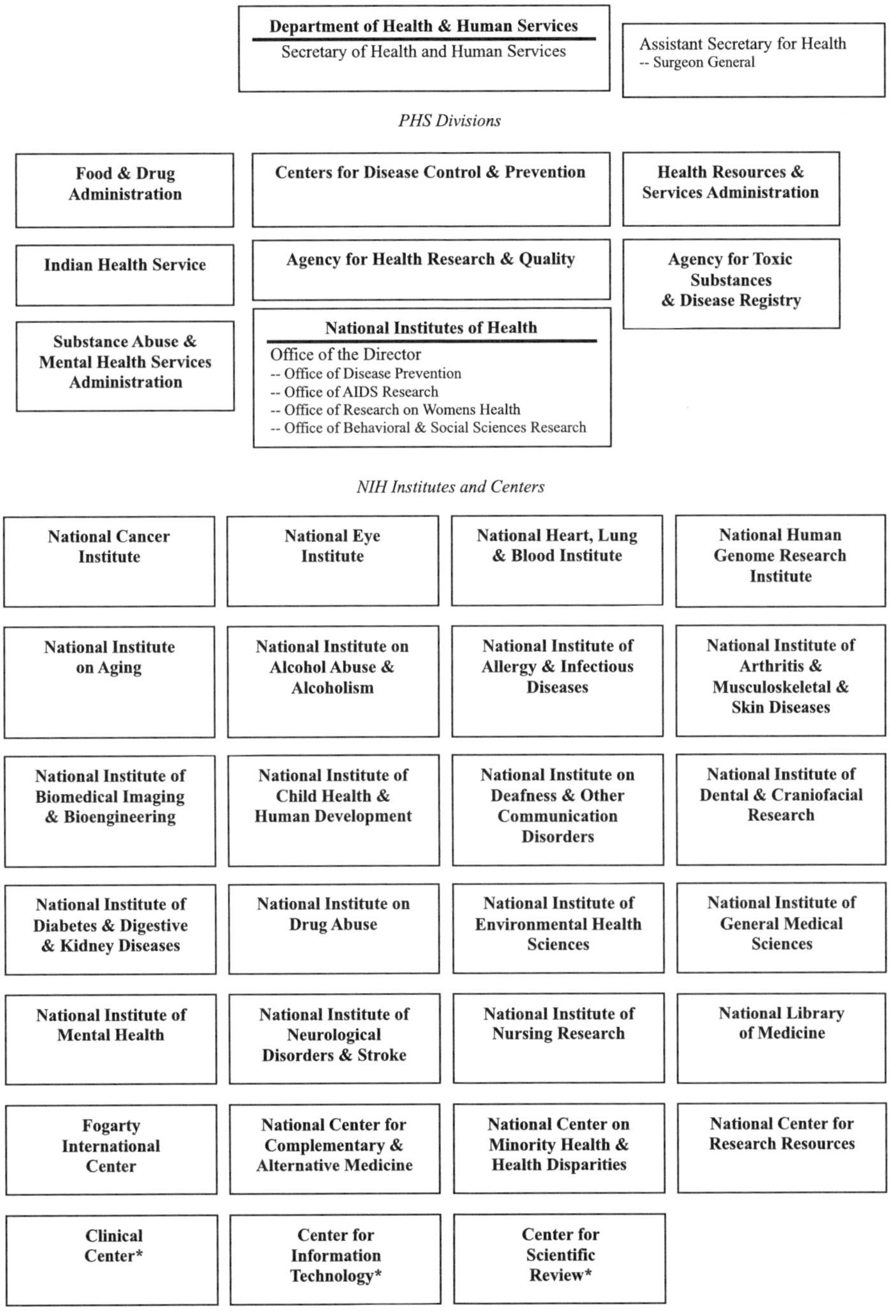

The Evolution of NIH's Organizational Structure

Department of Health & Human Services
Secretary of Health and Human Services

Assistant Secretary for Health
-- Surgeon General

PHS Divisions

Food & Drug Administration	Centers for Disease Control & Prevention	Health Resources & Services Administration
Indian Health Service	Agency for Health Research & Quality	Agency for Toxic Substances & Disease Registry
Substance Abuse & Mental Health Services Administration	**National Institutes of Health** Office of the Director -- Office of Disease Prevention -- Office of AIDS Research -- Office of Research on Womens Health -- Office of Behavioral & Social Sciences Research	

NIH Institutes and Centers

National Cancer Institute	National Eye Institute	National Heart, Lung & Blood Institute	National Human Genome Research Institute
National Institute on Aging	National Institute on Alcohol Abuse & Alcoholism	National Institute of Allergy & Infectious Diseases	National Institute of Arthritis & Musculoskeletal & Skin Diseases
National Institute of Biomedical Imaging & Bioengineering	National Institute of Child Health & Human Development	National Institute on Deafness & Other Communication Disorders	National Institute of Dental & Craniofacial Research
National Institute of Diabetes & Digestive & Kidney Diseases	National Institute on Drug Abuse	National Institute of Environmental Health Sciences	National Institute of General Medical Sciences
National Institute of Mental Health	National Institute of Neurological Disorders & Stroke	National Institute of Nursing Research	National Library of Medicine
Fogarty International Center	National Center for Complementary & Alternative Medicine	National Center on Minority Health & Health Disparities	National Center for Research Resources
Clinical Center*	Center for Information Technology*	Center for Scientific Review*	

*These centers do not make research grants.

FIGURE 2.1 Current Organization of NIH Institutes

by life stage have complex relationships to those organized by disease group or organ system with extensive overlap with the missions of other institutes; for example, the National Institute of Child Health and Human Development (NICHD) overlaps in nearly all of its research with other categorical institutes and in many ways serves as an institute for the profession of pediatric research and, to some extent, obstetrics research. Such overlaps can create tensions among institutes— some that are likely to be beneficial and some that are likely to be detrimental, depending on how they are acknowledged and responded to.

The most common mechanism of origin of the institutes has been the congressional mandate responding to the health advocacy community. Some, however, have developed in their own special circumstances. The National Human Genome Research Institute was established by NIH around a particular scientific objective. NIEHS, which focuses on the health effects of environmental exposures, was organized around a health problem, but not at the urging of health advocacy groups. NICHD and the National Institute on Aging (NIA) were organized around population groups (in 1962 and 1974); more recently, units focused on the health of women and minority groups were established in the 1990s and may be candidates for eventual elevation to institute status. The National Institute of Nursing Research was organized around a professional group—nurses—in 1993, and the establishment of the National Institute of Biomedical Imaging and Bioengineering (NIBIB) was authorized in 2000 after a 5-year advocacy campaign by radiologists and bioengineers.

Each institute except for the National Cancer Institute (NCI) has a director with a research background who is appointed by the Secretary of Health and Human Services. (The director of NCI was made a presidential appointee by the National Cancer Act of 1971; see Box 2A.) Each institute has a national advisory council to advise the institute director on policies and priorities and to provide a second level of review for extramural grant applications recommended for funding. All but one of those councils are appointed by the Secretary of Health and Human Services. (The National Cancer Advisory Board and the President's Cancer Panel of NCI are appointed by the President.) All institutes but one (the National Institute of General Medical Sciences) have intramural programs that perform basic and clinical research at the Clinical Center, in laboratory facilities on the NIH Bethesda campus, or elsewhere. Boards of Scientific Counselors advise each institute director on and oversee the performance of the intramural program and its researchers. Until recently, each director had a staff that mirrored the staff of the NIH director, including deputies for intramural and extramural research and offices for budget, administration, communications, legislation, and personnel. (Some of these functions have been or may be consolidated under the One HHS initiative discussed below.) The extramural grant programs of the institutes receive the largest share of their budgets. As measured by their budgets, institutes have grown at different rates over time. Starting from a small base, new institutes tend to receive large percentage budget increases in their early years.

> **Box 2A**
> **The National Cancer Act of 1971 [P.L. 92-218]**
>
> - Outgrowth of the report of the National Panel of Consultants on the conquest of cancer (the Yarborough Commission)
> - Elevated and expanded certain authorities of the National Cancer Institute director, including appointment by the President and preparation and submission of the annual budget estimate (Bypass Budget) directly to the President
> - Established the President's Cancer Panel and the National Cancer Advisory Board
> - Initiated the National Cancer Program under Sec. 407 of the PHS Act as follows: "(a) The director of the National Cancer Institute shall coordinate all of the activities of the National Institutes of Health relating to cancer with the National Cancer Program. (b) In carrying out the National Cancer Program, the director of the National Cancer Institute shall: (1) With the advice of the National Cancer Advisory Board, plan and develop an expanded, intensified, and coordinated cancer research program encompassing the programs of the National Cancer Institute, related programs of the other research institutes, and other Federal and non-Federal programs."
> - Authorized the first cancer centers
> - Established cancer control programs as necessary for cooperation with state and other health agencies
> - Established an information dissemination program
> - Established the International Cancer Research Data Bank

CENTERS

There are two types of centers. Some do not fund or conduct research, but rather provide operational support to the rest of NIH. The Center for Scientific Review (CSR), for example, is concerned solely with coordinating the activities of the set of scientific peer review panels called study sections, which review and score applications submitted to NIH for research grants and fellowships and recommend the most promising ones to the institutes for funding. Other centers conduct or support research and have been established as a result of legislation, for example, the Fogarty International Center.

OFFICE OF THE DIRECTOR

To carry out responsibilities that include planning, coordinating, and managing the programs of the 27 institutes and centers, the NIH director is assisted by units in OD known collectively as OD Operations. In addition, several offices and programs in OD address problems that the director or Congress believe need high-level NIH-wide attention. In all, 12 staff offices and 4 program offices report to the Director,[4] in addition to the 27 institute and center directors.

---

[4] See OD organization chart at http://www1.od.nih.gov/oma/manualchapters/management/1123/nih.pdf and "Organization and Functions, NIH, OD" at http://odeo.od.nih.gov/about/org/tocodo~1.htm.

The 1980s and 1990s saw the development of program offices in OD to help to promote and coordinate activities that are not solely in the portfolios of any of the individual institutes (Table 2-1). The Office of Disease Prevention, which includes the Office of Rare Diseases (ORD), the Office of Dietary Supplements (ODS), and the Office of Medical Applications of Research, was created in 1985 as a response to a congressional desire to increase disease prevention research. It is headed by an associate director for disease prevention. The Office of AIDS Research was established in 1988 to coordinate AIDS research and is also headed by an associate director. The Office of Research on Women's Health and the Office of Behavioral and Social Sciences Research were created in 1990 and 1995, respectively. Two program offices also created in the 1990s (alternative medicine and minority health) have since been elevated to center status, which gives them national advisory councils and the authority to award research grants. The Office of Bioengineering and Bioimaging has become an institute, NIBIB. Funding for OAR is specified in the appropriation act, and the funding of several other offices is earmarked in the OD

TABLE 2.1 Current Program Offices in the Office of the Director

Office	Year Established	Major Focus
Office of AIDS Research	1988	Planning, coordination, evaluation, and funding of all NIH AIDS research and support of trans-NIH coordinating committees in areas of AIDS research
Office of Research on Women's Health	1990	Focal point for women's health research at NIH, including establishment of a research agenda; inclusion of women as participants in NIH-supported research; and support of women in biomedical careers
Office of Disease Prevention, which includes the Office of Rare Diseases (1993), Office of Dietary Supplements (1995), and Office of Medical Applications of Research (1977)	1985	Coordination of disease prevention activities, advice to director on disease prevention research; promotion and coordination of NIH-wide research on rare or orphan diseases and on the role of dietary supplements in health; work with institutes and centers to assess, translate, and disseminate results of biomedical research that can be used in delivery of health services
Office of Behavioral and Social Sciences Research	1995	Stimulation of behavioral and social science research throughout NIH and its integration with other research conducted or supported by NIH

appropriation in the conference committee report, for example, $10.4 million for ORD and $17.0 million for the ODS in FY 2002.

The NIH director reports directly to the Secretary of Health and Human Services. Although the NIH director has considerable influence with Congress and the Administration with respect to the overall budget of each institute and center, he or she does not have strong formal authority with respect to the operation of the institutes. Institute and center directors have considerable autonomy, but they probably recognize the benefits of having a strong NIH director in securing increased support from Congress and the administration. Ideally, the NIH director is not only a distinguished scientist and a person with compelling ideas, but also an able leader with the ability to recruit other effective leaders and work well with the Secretary of Health and Human Services, other members of the administration, and Congress. The director has a small ($10 million) discretionary fund and, in principle, the authority to transfer up to 1% of an institute's or center's appropriation to another unit as long as the transfer does not increase any one appropriation by more than 3%. The federal budget and appropriation process, which culminates in a set of appropriations to NIH and its various institutes and centers, is the most important management tool available to the NIH director, who may use it to influence priorities and ensure that NIH is responding to opportunities and problems as he or she sees them develop. The budget and appropriation process, which begins internally, ultimately involves substantial interaction with the Department of Health and Human Services (DHHS), the Office of Management and Budget (OMB), and, on rare occasions, the President. Because of the central and historically generous role of Congress in the appropriations process, health advocacy groups are most likely to direct their lobbying efforts at the legislature.

THE BUDGET PROCESS

To understand how NIH has evolved, it is important to understand its funding environment and budget process (see Figure 2.2). NIH's statutory authority comes from the Public Health Service Act (PHSA) of 1944, as amended (42 U.S.C., et seq.). Some institutes and several programs (training and facilities construction) are subject to time and dollar authorizations that require periodic renewal by Congress.[5] The last authorization, the NIH Revitalization Act of 1993, lapsed in 1996 (P.L. 103-43); the effort to renew the authorization in 1996 failed because of conflict over provisions about the use of fetal tissue in research. There have been no further efforts to pass a general reauthorization of NIH.[6]

---

[5] The War on Cancer Act of 1971 was the first to impose time and dollar limits on an institute.
[6] The 1994 authorization for the National Institute of Mental Health, the National Institute on Alcohol Abuse and Alcoholism, and the National Institute on Drug Abuse (P.L. 102-321) has also lapsed. See Congressional Budget Office, 2002.

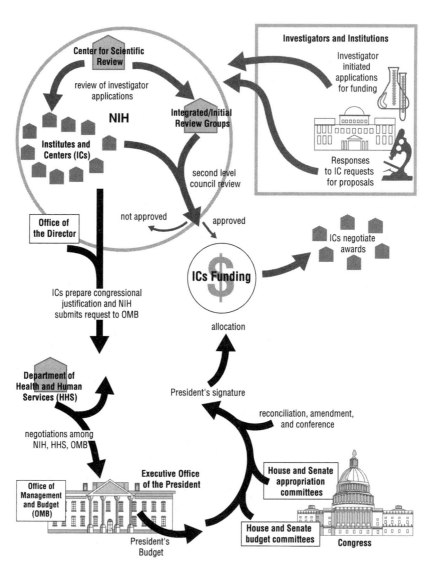

FIGURE 2.2 This figure illustrates the complex processes involved in NIH's budget. To begin the process, the institutes and centers work with the NIH director to develop their budget requests using guidance from OMB and HHS. The resulting budget is submitted through HHS and OMB to the President, and then appropriated by Congress, although numerous changes may be negotiated at many points along the way. After the institutes and centers receive their funding allocations, money is awarded to individual investigators and institutions through the peer review system under the administration of individual institutes and centers. Investigators may initiate proposals for funding on topics of their own choosing or may submit proposals in response to solicitations on specific topics from the institutes and centers.

Since 1996, NIH has operated on the basis of annual appropriation bills, although technically appropriations amounting to nearly half of NIH's funding are unauthorized. In the absence of authorizations, the appropriation committees, in their legislation and report language, have provided guidance that is similar to the guidance that authorizing committees enact. From time to time, bills to make specific changes in the PHSA are introduced; sometimes they are passed, such as the one that established NIBIB in 2000 (P.L. 106-580) and the one that established centers of excellence for research on the muscular dystrophies in 2001 (P.L. 107-84).

NIH, DHHS, OMB, and Congress manage the NIH appropriation primarily through a mechanism budget, that is, a set of budget functions that aggregate similar types of expenditures across NIH. Most of the budget (more than 80%) funds extramural activities, including research, training, and construction of facilities.[7]

Six congressional committees affect NIH funding: the authorizing and appropriating committees for DHHS in each house and the House and Senate Budget Committees. Officially, the budget committees set targets for NIH appropriations in the DHHS budget. The role of the authorizing committees is to set a level of funding that the appropriations committees may not exceed, although historically NIH has benefited from having an open-ended authorization, that is, Congress authorized "such sums as may be necessary" without a time limit. During a period of conflict between the President and Congress in the 1970s, Congress began to exert tighter control over some institutes by imposing time and dollar limits in the authorizing legislation. Currently, NCI, the National Heart, Lung, and Blood Institute, NIA, the National Institute of Mental Health (NIMH), the National Institute on Drug Abuse (NIDA), the National Institute on Alcohol Abuse and Alcoholism (NIAAA), NLM, and the National Research Service Awards (training and fellowship programs) are subject to time-and-dollar limits. As noted above, those programs have been operating with unauthorized appropriations since 1996, which underlines the fact that currently the appropriations committees exert the most influence on NIH. The authorizing committees can and do originate specific pieces of legislation affecting the organization of NIH, such as the law creating NIBIB. But the appropriations committees are not required to fund mandates in authorizing legislation.

The appropriations committees tend to have substantial influence on all aspects of NIH, including its organization, because of the rather open-ended grants of authority by the authorizing committees. Although they do not put much detail into law—usually just the total for each appropriation—they can use the reports that accompany bills to mandate NIH actions, including establishment of new organizational units. Report language does not have the force of law, but agencies try to

---

[7]The extramural share of the NIH budget is a little larger than the 80.9% accounted for by research grants, training awards, research and development contracts, and extramural construction in FY 2002 because the National Library of Medicine, Cancer Prevention and Control, and Office of the Director budgets also include some extramural support.

follow it because they know that they will be before the appropriations committees again each year.

The main impact of the congressional budget process on NIH has been to reinforce the autonomy of the institutes and centers through their separate appropriations. That means that the NIH director has no formal role in the budget *execution* stage, except for the seldom-used authority to transfer up to 1% of each institute's appropriation.

ADVISORY COMMITTEES

Like other federal science agencies, NIH makes extensive use of advisory committees (see Box 2B). The committees are composed of nonfederal scientists, health advocates, and laypersons to ensure that scientific expertise and public input are considered in making policies and evaluating programs. Advisory committees also foster a broader understanding of public concerns by the scientific community and increase public understanding of the scientific and technical impediments to research progress (NIH, 2001). NIH had over 140 chartered advisory committees as of May 2002—more than any other federal agency.[8] In total these advisory groups have 4,298 members, of whom 75% are members of the scientific review groups that evaluate applications for research funding. All the groups operate under the guidelines of the Federal Advisory Committee Act of 1972, as amended.

NIH uses advisory committees for initial and second-level peer review of applications for research grants and for policy and program advice. The overall purpose of the committees is to help to ensure that NIH programs are responsive to both scientific opportunity and health needs. The system of advisory committees is also an important mechanism for coordination and management. They include the Advisory Committee to the Director (ACD), the director's Council of Public Representatives (COPR), and the advisory councils established by law for each institute. The director's level advisory groups and ad hoc groups appointed to address particular issues provide NIH leaders with external views and advice on overall research needs and program priorities. The national advisory councils to the institutes, which include scientists and laypeople, provide a similar function to institute directors.

PEER REVIEW SYSTEM

If the institutes and centers are the public face of NIH, the study sections and peer review system are its scientific face. The fact that the research proposed by extramural scientists must pass muster with experts in their field and that all extramural awards, which account for more than 80% of NIH expenditures, are peer reviewed has been and continues to be central to NIH's success. The peer review

---

[8]See overview and list of committees by appointing officials at http://www1.od.nih.gov/cmo/about/index.html.

Box 2B
NIH Advisory Committees

NIH uses four types of advisory committees. Two are directly involved in reviewing grant applications, through what NIH calls a "dual review system."

Integrated/Initial Review Groups and **Special Emphasis Panels**—provide scientific and technical merit review which is the *first* level of peer review of research grant applications and contract proposals. These groups can be located in CSR or created and used by individual institutes who choose not to use CSR for review of particular initiatives. Within CSR, these groups comprise the study sections.

National Advisory Councils and Boards—perform the *second* level of peer review for research grant applications and offer advice and recommendations on policy and program development, program implementation, evaluation, and other matters of significance to the mission and goals of the respective institutes or centers. They also provide oversight of research conducted by each institute's or center's intramural program.

Thus, in the first level of review, grant applications are peer-reviewed by the integrated/initial review groups and the special emphasis panels primarily for their scientific value and technical merit. In the second level of review, grant applications are reviewed by a national advisory council (or board), which is composed of both scientists and lay representatives noted for their active involvement and expertise in an area of health. The council recommends applications for funding to the institute (or center) director based not only on scientific merit but also on the relevance of the proposed project to the institute's mission and priorities.

The dual review system, which separates the scientific assessment of proposed projects from policy decisions about scientific areas to be supported and the level of resources to be allocated, permits a more objective evaluation than would result from a single level of review. The dual system of review provides the responsible NIH officials with the best available advice about scientific as well as societal values and needs (NIH, 1992b).[a]

The two other types of advisory bodies are:

Boards of Scientific Counselors—review and evaluate the research programs and investigators of the *intramural* laboratories.

Program Advisory Committees—provide advice on specific research programs, future research needs and opportunities, and identify and evaluate extramural initiatives.

The President appoints two committees: the National Cancer Advisory Board and the President's Cancer Panel. The secretary of HHS appoints 32 committees, including the national advisory councils of the institutes and centers, Board of Regents of NLM, the ACD, and the Office of AIDS Research advisory council. The NIH director appoints 74, although about half of them are the initial review groups and special emphasis panels in CSR and the institutes and centers. The director also appoints advisory committees to program offices in OD (except OAR), boards of scientific counselors (except NCI), COPR, and for certain research areas (e.g., sickle cell disease, sleep disorders, recombinant DNA, medical rehabilitation research). Some are appointed by institute directors, especially the NCI director under the authority of the National Cancer Act of 1971.

The President generally follows the recommendations of the secretary of Health and Human Services in appointing advisory committee members, and the Secretary generally follows the advice of the NIH and institute directors in filling positions, although they add their own candidates from time to time. During the 1972-1974 period, when the Nixon Administration was trying to exert greater control over the NIH budget, there was a great deal of conflict with the scientific community over the perceived politicization of the advisory committee appointment process. This issue re-emerges from time to time, and is of current concern.

---

[a]Contracts are subjected to a similar peer review process, except the second level of review is by senior institute staff.

system is not perfect but it is the best guarantee we have that scientists will carry out research that is of high quality and has high potential for scientific progress. The state of scientific understanding and the potential for near-term progress are always difficult to assess and may vary considerably across disciplines and diseases. At any given time, some areas of research are riper for progress than others. The interaction of the two systems—institute-based assessment of need on the one hand and the study section/peer review system on the other—enables NIH to reconcile the sometimes conflicting goals of addressing the most important health needs through research and funding the best science. Although the categorical nature of the institutes helps policy makers to allocate funding among broad areas of health research (such as cancer, heart disease, arthritis, brain disorders, child development, and genomics), the structure and process of peer review are intended to ensure that research that is likely to be the most productive is funded.

The intramural program uses a retrospective process for reviewing the research of NIH's own scientists rather than the prospective peer review described above. The intramural program has been the subject of several reviews (Institute of Medicine, 1988; NIH, 1994).

CSR was established in 1946 to administer the review and evaluation of proposals for the rapidly expanding grant program, and peer review has been the centerpiece of this operation. Like institutes and centers, study sections established by CSR proliferated over the years, from 20 in 1946 to more than 100 in 1994, plus many ad hoc and special emphasis panels. By that time, it became apparent that the peer review system needed restructuring to respond to changes in the way science is conducted. According to CSR, more and more applications address complex biological problems with broad, multidisciplinary research programs that are collaborative, multi-investigator, and multi-center, thus calling for a greater breadth of expertise. "There are also more trans-NIH initiatives that involve extensive collaborations within and across disciplines and institutions. The CSR peer review system, designed many years ago with a focus on individual investigator-initiated research, may no longer provide the one size that fits all. More flexible ways of operation are likely required...." (CSR, 1999 and 2000a).

By the mid-1990s, pressure for a comprehensive reexamination of the structure of the study sections and the organization of CSR had grown. In 1998, the Panel on Scientific Boundaries for Review recommended a substantial change in the structure of review groups. The panel suggested that as much science as possible be reviewed on an organ-system or disease basis, rather than discipline-related study sections. It called for grouping study sections into 24 clusters called Integrated Review Groups (IRGs), most of them addressing basic, translational, and clinical research within the context of the biological problem being addressed, such as a particular disease or physiological function (CSR, 2000b).[9]

---

[9] See the CSR website for detailed information about the restructuring of CSR and the peer review process at http://www.csr.nih.gov/about.htm. Also at http://www.nih.gov/archives/renamed.htm.

This recommendation acknowledges the advent of molecular medicine, where biochemistry, genetics, molecular and cellular biology have become tools applied to virtually all fields of health-related research. Molecular medicine applications will be reviewed in the context of the biological questions addressed rather than lumped in discipline-related study sections where they will compete against each other."(CSR, 2000c).

The panel also recommended IRGs for basic scientific discovery and methods development not associated with a particular disease, and clusters addressing cross-cutting fields such as aging and development. Of the 24 IRGs, 7 were recently reorganized and will be retained as is, 6 will be new, and 11 will be modified from existing IRGs.[10]

In addition, when the Alcohol, Drug Abuse, and Mental Health Administration's three institutes—NIHM, NIDA, and NIAAA— were reintegrated into NIH in 1993, the number of institutes with large neuro- and behavioral science research portfolios increased to five. This necessitated the complete restructuring of neuroscience and behavioral science review in 1996, which involved substantial participation by the extramural research community.

In the second phase of the restructuring, which began in February 2001, external advisory teams were brought in to assess and recommend changes in the study group structure of each IRG.[11] Currently there are 159 study sections, an average of 8, but ranging from 3 to 12, per IRG. After the process of reviewing and restructuring the study sections is completed in 2003, ad hoc external advisory groups will review each IRG every 5 years. Periodic evaluation is intended to keep the structure of study sections current with the changing landscape of science and is an important development. If the plan for regular review is carried forward, it should prevent the need for a major overhaul in the future of the kind that is being undertaken by CSR at present. The Committee commends NIH for proceeding with these ongoing reforms.

HISTORICAL FORCES BEHIND ORGANIZATIONAL COMPLEXITY

The establishment of NCI in 1937 began the long history of creating categorical institutes that organized research in the context of particular diseases. Citizen advocacy for NIH funding and growth grew in scale and sophistication after World War II and changed national health policy. The wartime experiences of leading government scientists and the success of the Office of Scientific Research and Development brought about wide acceptance of a broad federal role in supporting research in our nation's universities. In addition, military recruitment and mobilization produced greater recognition of the roles of health and disease in determining

---

[10]See http://www.csr.nih.gov/events/implementplan.htm.
[11]As of May 16, 2002, meetings had been held and proposed guidelines posted for 10 IRGs at http://www.csr.nih.gov/PSBR/IRGComments.htm.

the physical fitness of American military personnel. For example, during the early 1940s about 21% of the 2 million potential military recruits could not meet Selective Service dental requirements. This observation led President Truman to sign legislation that created the National Institute of Dental Research (NIDR) on June 24, 1948. At that time, NIH consisted of three institutes—cancer, heart, and dental.

From the middle 1940s to 1974, health advocates were successful in persuading Congress to establish additional institutes, often against the wishes of administrations, which generally opposed creation of new categorical institutes. Elizabeth Drew (1967) described the interactions among the NIH leadership, congressional committees, and voluntary health associations. The philanthropist Mary Lasker, her associates, Florence Mahoney and Mike Gorman, and her friends in the medical research community, including Sidney Farber and Michael DeBakey, played an enormous facilitating role. Drew called Lasker, Mahoney, and their allies "noble conspirators."

Substantial post-Watergate changes in the political organization of Congress in the 1970s changed the relationships between the executive and legislative branches and marked a new era in activism generally. Congress assumed more oversight of executive agency programs—an oversight that often resulted in highly specific instructions regarding organizational details. The changes in Congress also eroded the traditional strong roles of committee chairs and dispersed power to subcommittee chairs and members. That enabled the health advocacy groups to lobby more widely and successfully for the creation of new organizational units at NIH.

In the 1980s, mass advocacy techniques pioneered by AIDS activists inspired other groups to organize at the grass roots as well as at the national level, creating an even more effective way to influence politicians in Washington. Some of the groups have continued the long established pattern of pushing for creation of named entities at NIH to create focal points for developing more research funding for particular diseases. That has often resulted in the establishment by Congress of a named program at the office level. Through continued pressure, offices may then be elevated to centers and, in some cases, to institute status. In addition, the practice of pressing for increased funding for specific diseases in existing institute programs, such as Parkinson's and Alzheimer's, became more prevalent in the 1990s.

Public need and scientific opportunity are not necessarily compatible or congruent. In the face of good intentions, some consider it risky to invest in research on a disease if the science is not ready and the ability to make progress is unclear. It is possible to argue that the tension between disease-based advocacy and scientific opportunity has been productive and has led to more funding for basic research while making scientists more sensitive to public expectations of reducing the burden of disease by investing tax dollars in research. Achieving the appropriate balance between need and opportunity is difficult, however, and results in understandable tensions among the scientific community, health advocacy groups, NIH management, the Executive Branch, and Congress about who should determine NIH priorities.

Over the last 25 years, the scientific community—largely through professional and university associations—has also become a part of the dynamic that drives the growth of the NIH budget. As a result, the political environment has become a quadrilateral relationship among scientific associations, voluntary health organizations, Congress, and administrations—all with an interest in improving health through research. But they do not always agree on how, or on how much relative to other national needs. The activism of scientific societies generally focuses on appropriations and on specific programs or problems, such as the need for informatics support or specific fundamental research initiatives. The scientific societies have generally opposed the creation of new units and pressed for increasing the numbers and amounts of grant awards, training programs, and improvements in the operation of the study section system.

NIH AND THE DEPARTMENT OF HEALTH AND HUMAN SERVICES

During the course of the Committee's work, several other independent activities focusing on administrative aspects of NIH were underway, most of which are related to NIH's responsibilities as an agency of DHHS.

Over its history, NIH has rarely been directed to add new organizational units by an administration. Indeed, most often DHHS, OMB, and other parts of the Executive Office of the President oppose creating new institutes and centers, and OMB, in its institutional oversight role, usually attempts to enforce this. At the departmental level, the same desire to rationalize and order the subcomponents of the department apply. Over the years, DHHS secretaries and NIH directors have generally not favored expansion.

Given this history, it is not surprising that DHHS Secretary Tommy Thompson has issued instructions to consolidate administrative functions, such as personnel management, communications, congressional liaison, and travel, throughout DHHS. The "One HHS" initiative has the stated goal of better integrating DHHS management functions across its operating and staff divisions. The initiative has already resulted in consolidation of some administrative functions. Although all the operating divisions of DHHS are involved, NIH is especially affected because of its highly decentralized structure. Of 40 personnel offices in DHHS, for example, NIH previously accounted for 27. These have now been consolidated into one for NIH and three for the rest of the department (DHHS, 2001).[12]

Plans to consolidate the communications, legislative, and congressional affairs offices of NIH have been only partly carried out because of objections from Congress. Many of those offices, which focus on outreach to the public and Congress, were established in the institutes and centers by statute and therefore may be less subject to departmental consolidation policies. DHHS has plans for consolidating other functions at NIH, such as budgeting, finance, and procurement, and is encour-

---

[12]The plan contains several principles, including "managing HHS as one department."

aging NIH to consider outsourcing some of its administrative functions (for example, grants management), citing the goals of the President's Management Agenda (OMB, 2002). Late in its deliberations, the Committee chair was able to meet with DHHS officials to discuss centralization. Also in early 2003, the House Energy and Commerce Committee and the House Oversight and Investigations Subcommittee initiated examinations of how NIH manages and polices its research portfolio, particularly how it reviews and manages grants (Ochs, 2003).

While the Committee believes that it is critical for initiatives to eliminate inefficiencies to continue, centralization of administrative functions is not always the most effective way of proceeding, especially when these functions are difficult to separate from the performance of the primary mission (Sclar, 2000). It would not serve anyone's interests if well meaning efforts to increase efficiency undermined the effectiveness of NIH's programs and its ability to recruit talented leaders at all levels. Assembling the Nation's best talent to work on the biomedical frontier is both very challenging and a qualitatively different operation than hiring for more routine and common administrative tasks. The Committee believes that initiatives to centralize or outsource from NIH key science-related functions, such as aspects of grants management, fail to appreciate how closely this so-called administrative function is tied to NIH's primary mission. Treating crucial science management functions as general administrative services could do great harm to the NIH research enterprise. Moreover, the Committee finds the prospect of mandatory centralization of some administrative aspects of NIH's scientific mission contrary to a stated intent of the President's Management Agenda (OMB, 2002), which is "Freedom to Manage":

> Federal managers are greatly limited in how they can use available financial and human resources to manage programs; they lack much of the discretion given to their private sector counterparts to do what it takes to get the job done. Red tape still hinders the efficient operation of government organizations; excessive control and approval mechanisms afflict bureaucratic processes. Micro-management from various sources—Congressional, departmental, and bureau—imposes unnecessary operational rigidity.

Recommendation 1: *Centralization of Management Functions*
Any efforts to consolidate or centralize management functions at NIH, either within NIH or at the DHHS level, should be considered only after careful study of circumstances unique to NIH and its successes in carrying out its research and training mission. A structured and studied approach should be used to assure that centralization will not undermine NIH's ability to identify, fund, and manage the best research and training proposals and programs in support of improving health.

In response to DHHS and OMB administrative efforts to reduce duplication and overlap and to ensure resource redirection toward mission-critical areas, NIH senior management announced the formation of the NIH Administrative Restructuring Advisory Committee in April 2003. The Advisory Committee will include broad NIH representation and focus on trans-NIH proposals to change NIH administrative management functions (NIH, 2003a). The Committee believes that NIH is being responsive to justifiable concerns about improved efficiencies and encourages DHHS to work with the NIH Advisory Committee as it conducts its work.

NIH'S LOCATION IN THE FEDERAL GOVERNMENT

The Committee also briefly discussed one other recurrent issue surrounding NIH's place in the Executive Branch. Since 1952, NIH has been housed in the equivalent of DHHS. However, as the structure of the department has changed and as NIH's budget and prominence have grown, the appropriateness of NIH's placement has been questioned by some. NIH is now responsible for over 50% of federal nondefense R&D expenditures. Moreover, other large science-supporting agencies, such as the National Science Foundation (NSF) and the National Aeronautics and Space Administration, enjoy independent agency status. That status enables them to interact more directly with the leadership of the Executive Branch, including OMB and the rest of the Executive Office of the President, and with appropriate committees of Congress. Some argue that the fact that NIH is subsumed in DHHS and therefore unable to have such direct interactions potentially compromises its ability to carry out its mission most expeditiously and effectively.

Those who oppose making NIH independent of DHHS argue that it is important to keep NIH embedded in the department because the NIH mission of health research is an integral part of the DHHS mission and is analogous to the arrangement in other departments, such as the co-location of the Defense Advanced Research Projects Agency and other defense R&D organizations with the service organizations in DOD. Independent agency status for NIH would also risk eroding the strong political support that it enjoys in Congress and among the voluntary health organizations and might upset the productive relationships that exist among NIH's various constituencies, which may be very difficult to reestablish under new circumstances. Furthermore, many feel that NIH needs more, not less, connection with the Food and Drug Administration, the Centers for Disease Control and Prevention, and other PHS agencies.

Although not clearly in the purview of this study, the issue of NIH's location in the Executive Branch was raised by a few people during the Committee's deliberations. The concern deserves more extensive consideration than could be provided by this Committee.

SUMMARY

NIH is a distinctive organization that is best thought of as a federation of units tied together by common processes and overall objectives. The processes are those for deploying federal research funding across a wide array of institutions and individuals to mobilize the nation's best scientific capabilities to focus on NIH's priorities. The overall objectives are to advance the scientific frontier and to support research training in fields of special relevance to the nation's health needs.

Despite the similar processes and shared goal of its components, however, NIH is highly decentralized, and its priorities are influenced by a wide variety of key constituencies concerned with health and the vitality of the nation's biomedical research and development system. As a result, NIH's scientific portfolio is spread across a very large number of topics and fields among which it may be difficult to discern overall strategic goals or distinctive functions.

In chapters 4 through 6, the Committee addresses the implications of this highly decentralized structure both in terms of the strengths it brings to certain endeavors and the obstacles it can raise for others. The next chapter addresses the changing landscape for biomedical research and how this might affect NIH's organizational structure.

3

New Opportunities, New Challenges: The Changing Nature of Biomedical Science

The frontier of biomedical science has rarely been as exciting and as full of spectacular opportunities as it is today. From basic science through clinical research to health services research, the opportunities made available through the impressive advances of recent decades in the biomedical as well as the physical, computational, and behavioral and social sciences have brought us to a frontier of unprecedented opportunity. Those developments have also begun to transform the conduct of both large- and small-scale biological and biomedical research in rather dramatic ways. Although traditionally structured laboratory and clinical investigations are still its most essential components, several technical and scientific breakthroughs have altered how research is conducted. For example, high-throughput technologies are enabling rapid accumulation of unprecedented amounts of biological and health-related information. Nucleic acid and protein databases are revolutionizing some of the ways in which the structure and function of biomolecules and cells are studied. Databases and biological repositories have become ever more essential resources for scientists, and biocomputing and bioinformatics are indispensable tools in new types of investigations that are based on these vast amounts of data. Moreover, in some fields the scientific enterprise is characterized by the increased importance of large-scale and complex projects. All those additions to the traditional research paradigm are placing new demands on approaches to research funding and management because some parts of the scientific frontier require the creation of larger-scale products, significant new infrastructure investments,[1] or the mobilization of inter-

---

[1] At the same time that the present committee was conducting its work, the National Cancer Policy Board of the National Academies was preparing a report, *Large-Scale Biomedical Science: Exploring*

disciplinary research teams, sometimes involving large numbers of investigators at many institutions. More strategic planning and coordination of investigators on the part of the National Institutes of Health (NIH) as a whole are required if it is to make the most effective use of its resources.

Increasingly, investigators will need to integrate knowledge gained from high-throughput molecular research and high-powered imaging studies with knowledge from population-based epidemiological studies and clinical trials to learn what works and what does not work, what is safe and what is not safe. It seems clear, for example, that there will be a greater need for research on interactions among genetic variation, cell dynamics and behavioral, metabolic, nutritional, environmental, and pharmaceutical variables. And greater prominence must be given to research in the behavioral and social sciences, to health services research that is related to the more effective treatment of diseases and improvement of quality of life, and to the continuing evaluation of preventive interventions. Growing awareness of the association between socioeconomic status and health and health disparities provides new challenges as well as opportunities for research. The opportunities and needs raise the issues of setting research priorities and defining appropriate boundaries for NIH research, but they also raise questions about whether NIH's current institutional structure facilitates or limits the adaptability of its programs.

Finally, international and economic factors are changing the nature of science. First, a greater sense of urgency permeates some fields of research, given the threat of bioterrorism, persistent and emerging infectious diseases, and the complexity of the international environment for science with its pressing health needs. Second, private industry and foreign governments have substantially increased their funding of biomedical research and development (R&D) (National Science Foundation, 2002). Third, the increasingly global nature of science raises new challenges to the NIH structure with respect to international collaboration, capacity-building, and training.

An overview of how biomedical science has developed in the last decade and where it might be leading is helpful in determining whether NIH's current organizational structure is best suited to address emerging scientific opportunities and partner effectively with other federal agencies and the private sector. This chapter presents a snapshot of certain aspects of the current research environment with some speculation as to how it is changing.

CLINICAL RESEARCH NEEDS

Clinical research informs and stimulates fundamental science; conversely, basic laboratory and epidemiological research inform and stimulate clinical research. As

---

Strategies for Future Research (Institute of Medicine, 2003a). Some of the material in this chapter was gathered by the National Cancer Policy Board during its deliberations.

defined broadly by NIH in a report of a task force chaired by David G. Nathan (National Institutes of Health, 1997a),[2] clinical research includes

- Research conducted with human subjects or on material of human origin (tissues, specimens, and cognitive phenomena) in which an investigator interacts directly with human subjects. This research includes mechanisms of human disease, therapeutic interventions, clinical trials, and development of new technologies.
- Epidemiologic and behavioral studies.
- Outcomes and health services research.

Others might define clinical research more broadly to include some aspects of drug screening, and development of diagnostics and gene therapy—all laboratory-based activities but nonetheless patient-focused forms of research.

The research community recognizes a social compact with the public to help improve health by advancing knowledge along all relevant parts of the scientific frontier. At the same time, the translation of discoveries in fundamental and applied science into useful clinical and public health interventions and uses of such interventions to reduce disability, morbidity, and health disparities are the ways the public measures the success of its investments in biological and behavioral research.

Yet for nearly 25 years there have been persistent concerns about the health and future of our national efforts in clinical research (Wyngaarden, 1979). Reviews of its status and recommendations for improvement have been conducted previously and in a far more thorough manner than could this Committee. Most recently, the NIH director's Panel on Clinical Research was commissioned in the spring of 1995 by Harold Varmus, the director of NIH, because the "perception of crisis in clinical research that had simmered for decades had intensified by a funding shortage induced by managed care and new restrictions on the Federal budget" (National Institutes of Health, 1997a). More recently, members of the Clinical Research Roundtable of IOM published a review of the challenges facing the national clinical research enterprise (Sung et al., 2003).

NIH sponsors a large set of programs in clinical research and training through its institutes' and centers' extramural and intramural research programs; the agency is the largest sponsor of clinical research in the world. NIH spent $7.6 billion on clinical research in FY 2002, estimates it will spend $8.4 billion of its $27 billion budget in FY 2003 and projects spending $8.7 billion in FY 2004. A large portion of the clinical research supported by NIH occurs extramurally in hospitals and clinics affiliated with medical schools, independent research institutes, and health departments throughout the United States. A smaller but vitally important portion

---

[2]NIH's definition excludes in vitro studies that use human tissues but do not deal directly with patients. That is, clinical, or patient-oriented, research is research in which it is necessary to know the identity of the patient from whom the cells or tissues under study are derived.

of NIH's clinical research portfolio is conducted through the intramural research programs of the institutes and at its Clinical Center.

The clinical research programs sponsored by NIH differ from most of those supported by the private sector in that NIH-sponsored clinical research focuses most heavily on increased understanding of disease prevalence, disease mechanisms, and long-term outcomes of therapies. Appropriately, most clinical research sponsored by the private sector (such as pharmaceutical, biotechnology, and medical device companies) focuses on testing the efficacy and safety of new drugs and devices before their approval by the Food and Drug Administration (FDA). Both types of clinical research are essential to advance human health, and they depend on one another.

Clinical research is often conducted on a large-scale at multiple institutions across the country or even around the world. For example, in 1991, NIH launched the Women's Health Initiative (WHI) with the broad goal of investigating strategies for the prevention and control of some of the most common causes of morbidity and mortality among postmenopausal women, including cancers, cardiovascular disease, and osteoporotic fractures.[3] Congress provided special funding, totaling $213 million over 4 years, through the Office of the Director. The WHI has functioned as a trans-NIH consortium and is one of the largest studies of its kind ever undertaken in the United States, involving more than 40 centers nationwide and 162,000 women. The first results from the WHI have been reported, for example, the rates of cancers, heart disease, and osteoporosis in women taking hormone replacement therapy (Pradhan et al., 2002). The findings have had a large and prompt impact on medical practice and on the ways physicians prescribe such therapy for their patients.

Another example is the Collaborative Programs of Excellence in Autism, launched in 1997.[4] At the request of Congress, NIH formed the Autism Coordinating Committee (ACC) to enhance the quality, pace, and coordination of NIH efforts to find a cure for autism, and the ACC has been instrumental in the research into, understanding of, and advances in autism. Five institutes (the National Institute of Child Health and Human Development, National Institute of Environmental Health Sciences, National Institute of Mental Health (NIMH), National Institute of Neurological Disorders and Stroke, and National Institute on Deafness and Communication Disorders) are members of the ACC. In addition, representatives of the National Institute of Allergy and Infectious Diseases and the National Center for Complementary and Alternative Medicine participate in ACC meetings, as do representatives of the Centers for Disease Control and Prevention (CDC), FDA, and the US Department of Education.

Because many major diseases have common risk factors, broad-based, potentially large-scale, and trans-NIH projects are sometimes required to share information and show linkages more precisely. For example, smoking, high-fat and

---

[3] See http://www.nhlbi.nih.gov/health/public/heart/other/whi/wmn_hlt.htm.
[4] See http://www.nichd.nih.gov/autism/nihacc.cfm.

low-fiber diets, physical inactivity, and exposures to exogenous and endogenous toxins are all likely to contribute to the development and progression of numerous diseases that are within the purview of multiple institutes. But despite a growing list of successful trans-NIH collaborations, NIH officials told the Committee that NIH has for decades had a notably difficult time in funding clinical, let alone population-based, studies that involve major diseases that belong to multiple institutes, such as cancers, heart disease, pregnancy outcomes, and duodenal ulcers related to smoking. In addition to studies of causation, trials seeking reduction of lung cancer and heart disease with other agents (such as beta-carotene in the 1980s and 1990s and other antioxidants now) have been difficult to fund across institutes.[5] Generally, one institute has had to be willing to fund the whole study, but this often results in less than fully efficient investigations of diseases that fall outside the institute's mandate (such as heart disease in trials supported by NCI or cancer in trials supported by NHLBI) or in passing up the opportunity to broaden the benefit of a trial at a modest cost.

Evidence-Based Medicine and Health Services Research

An increasingly important extension of the value of clinical trials is in research to enhance evidence-based medicine, which aims to take the best available information from clinical trials and observational studies and apply it in clinical practice. For example, despite a rich evidence base for management of cardiovascular disorders, study after study has demonstrated disconcertingly low rates of compliance with widely disseminated evidence-based treatment guidelines for managing such common cardiovascular conditions as coronary heart disease, congestive heart failure, and high blood pressure. The difficulty in translating the results of clinical trials into clinical practice suggests the presence of multiple barriers to implementation. Although there is substantial overlap, the barriers are in four general domains related to science, the health profession, the patient, and the health system. Even very well-designed randomized clinical trials may fail to examine all the relevant risk factors and patient and cultural variables.

Barriers related to the health profession include lack of knowledge of the best current evidence, time constraints, and the overriding desire to avoid iatrogenic complications. Patient-related barriers include managing multiple prescriptions for multiple chronic conditions, time and financial constraints, and difficulties in engaging in health-modifying behaviors such as smoking cessation, exercise, and dietary modification. Barriers related to the health system include lack of sufficient insurance, lack of integrated approaches to the care of chronic illness, and the high cost of health care. The complexity of issues involved mandates a comprehensive and collaborative approach involving physicians and other health care professionals,

---

[5]These and related issues concerning trans-NIH initiatives were raised repeatedly during Committee interviews with NIH senior management.

patients and their families or other support systems, and the health care system itself if the myriad barriers to implementing evidence-based care are to be overcome (Rich, 2002). Indeed, much of the complexity is not fully understood and requires further research.

Health services research is within the mission of NIH. Some institutes, such as the National Institute on Aging, National Cancer Institute (NCI), NIMH, the National Institute on Drug Abuse, and the National Institute on Alcohol Abuse and Alcoholism, have substantial portfolios, even whole divisions, that focus specifically on health services research. Another Department of Health and Human Services agency, the Agency for Healthcare Research and Quality (AHRQ), takes the lead in some aspects of health services research and recommends strategies for monitoring and improving quality of care, but it cannot fully address the demand for the full array of such research. Furthermore, health services research is closely related at the disease or health-dimension level to treatment research, as well as to much more basic behavioral science (such as social psychology theory or organizational theory). Thus, there are many reasons to support health services research in multiple institutes. In fact, NIH estimates that it spends about $800 million per year on health services research compared with $300 million per year for the entire AHRQ budget (Sung et al., 2003; Helms, 2002). Clearly, more coordination across NIH and between NIH and other agencies, such as AHRQ, the Department of Veterans Affairs, and the Centers for Medicare and Medicaid Services, would advance this developing field.

INCREASING URGENCY IN SOME FIELDS OF RESEARCH

In the last few years, the United States has become increasingly and uncomfortably aware of its vulnerability to bioterrorist threats. Concerns about vaccine supplies, efficacy and safety of older vaccines, and the documentation for handling and storing materials that pose biological, chemical, and radioactive hazards have reopened discussions about public health research in general and about openness and secrecy in scientific communication (Omenn, 2003). The role of NIH in rapid response to research needs arising from bioterrorism—especially in areas where there is little incentive for private investment—has been the subject of recent analyses; some have questioned the agency's ability to be flexible and responsive (National Research Council, 2002).

New infectious diseases (West Nile virus and Severe Acute Respiratory Syndrome [SARS]) and reemerging infectious diseases (malaria in Virginia and tuberculosis worldwide), increasing antibiotic-resistance in pathogenic bacteria, and the threat of bioterrorism have caused renewed interest in infectious disease agents, epidemiology, and surveillance of potentially exposed populations (Omenn, 2003). Those research subjects require reaching across public health, agriculture, ecology, and other fields in ways that might not be typical or easy with NIH's current structural configuration. Beyond NIH, greater collaboration with the intelligence

community, emergency workers, law enforcement,
munications, and information industries will be
Council, 2002). The sudden spread of SARS in Ch
also highlights the need for rapid detection, identif
with CDC and international health organizations,
improving scientific knowledge of the coronavirus th
ing vaccines and treatments.

ADDRESSING HEALTH DISPARITIES

Increasing attention is being directed to the biological, genetic, and socioeconomic basis of health and whether all Americans are benefiting from health-related research advances. The life expectancy of members of many minority groups in the United States is still much shorter than that of white Americans. Recent years have seen gains in longevity and lessening of the impact of chronic diseases, but minority populations have not benefited as much as the white population. The disparities have many causes (Institute of Medicine, 2002).

The influence of racial bias is not limited to access to health care. Racial prejudice and discrimination can be sources of acute and chronic stress that have been linked to such conditions as cardiovascular disease and alcohol abuse (Cooper, 2001; Yen et al., 1999). Discrimination can restrict people's educational, employment, economic, residential, and partner choices, affecting health through pathways linked with what psychosocial scientists refer to as human capital. Environmental influences of industry, toxic waste disposal sites, and other geographic characteristics linked with poverty and minority status can result in serious disadvantages to minority groups' health (Institute of Medicine, 1999).

The increasingly recognized links among genetics, health, socioeconomic status, and macroeconomics emphasize the importance of research to examine and decrease the magnitude of health disparities. In 2000, the National Center on Minority Health and Health Disparities was established by the passage of the Minority Health and Health Disparities Research and Education Act of 2000 (PL 106-525), reflecting a concern among policymakers that NIH was not paying sufficient attention to this issue.[6]

THE GROWTH OF LARGE-SCALE AND DISCOVERY-DRIVEN SCIENCE

Most federally-supported biomedical research has been conducted through small independent projects initiated by individual investigators working in relatively small

---

[6]In particular, see July 26, 2000, hearing of the Senate Health, Education, Labor and Pensions Committee's Subcommittee on Public Health on health disparities of minorities, women, and underserved populations, and NIH's role in addressing them. Witnesses were also asked to comment on the proposed Health Care Fairness Act, S. 1880 and H.R. 3250.

research groups. Such research is typically hypothesis-driven, that is, aiming to address specific biological questions. That approach to research remains essential, but developments on the scientific frontier have encouraged scientists to consider also the increased importance of carefully selected broader and larger-scale projects, for example, to develop extensive pools of data and other research tools that can then facilitate the more conventional approach to research. This approach, often called "discovery" science, is based on the assumption that the analysis of a complete data set collected across the breadth of a biological system (for example, an entire genome) is likely to yield clues and patterns on which to base hypotheses about the relationships of important biomolecules operating in the system.

The Human Genome Project: An Important Additional Paradigm in Basic Biology

The biggest and most visible large-scale, discovery-driven research project in biology is the Human Genome Project (HGP), an international effort to map and sequence the entire human genome. When it was first proposed, many scientists opposed the project on the basis of its cost and size and the fact that it was managed science; they assumed it would take funding away from other, more important projects. It was also viewed by many as a forced transition away from hypothesis-driven science to a directed, hierarchical mode of "Big Science" (Cook-Deegan, 1994). Many argued that it was technically infeasible. Proponents of the HGP won out, especially as the Department of Energy began on its own, and NIH secured designated funds that allowed it to make its first awards in 1988. A draft sequence of the entire human genome was completed in 2000, and the full sequence in April 2003 (Pennisi, 2003). The data from the HGP constitute a vast and rich resource for biomedical research for many years to come.

The next challenge lies in identifying the functions of the genes and the complex regulatory dynamics of the cell to understand the mechanisms that lead to the creation of proteins and their functions (Burley, 2000). Sequences from the genome project are being analyzed with improved understanding of cell dynamics to help to identify protein families. Structural genomics uses computational analyses with structural determinations of the protein products to advance the study of protein function. Proteomics permits simultaneous examination of changes in expression levels and modifications of structure and function in health and disease. The resulting data must be assessed against a background of population-based studies entailing the generation, storage, and analysis of enormous quantities of epidemiologic, genotypic, and phenotypic data. The process of hunting for disease-related mechanisms that seem to be directly related to genetic material—once an expensive and arduous undertaking conducted by individual laboratories and investigators—has become rapid and highly automated; it is limited primarily by the incompleteness of our understanding of cell regulation, the unexpected complexity of many diseases, and the lack of a rich information base regarding many nongenetic risk factors in the relevant human populations. Despite the spectacular discoveries of recent decades there remain large gaps in our understanding of how genetic information is transformed into biological meaning. The challenge of this task has led some to warn of the prospect of a bottleneck between genome-based scientific advances and translation to clinical improvement (Nathan and Varmus, 2000).

The Mounting Importance of Biocomputing, Bioinformatics, and Clinical Informatics

As a result of the HGP, associated projects, and imaging research, biologists and clinical investigators are faced with more opportunity and data and a greater need to organize the data in a meaningful, coherent, and public manner than ever before. For example, automation has allowed fewer people to accomplish more sequencing in shorter periods. The immense amount of information generated by this class of projects is stimulating new collaborations among clinical medicine, biology, chemistry, physics, and the fields of bioinformatics, computer science, and mathematics. Large amounts of computational expertise are a necessity. To understand the similarities and differences among organisms of the same and different species, sophisticated comparisons must be conducted, and many of them cannot be conducted effectively solely with traditional tools. Using appropriately designed databases and powerful computers, bioinformatics is providing a view of the relationships among organisms that are sometimes separated in evolution by many millions of years. Computers can display patterns and periodicities that would rarely be found if searched for with traditional approaches and techniques (Hood, 2003). Thus, in many ways, biology is becoming an information science (Botstein, 2000). The creation and development of such databases and database technologies (methods for storing, retrieving, sharing, and analyzing biomedical data) are becoming more important in all biomedical fields. As more information from clinical trials becomes available, the need for standardization and interoperability of clinical databases will increase. Coordinating knowledge gained from a large and growing set of clinical trials with new insights from genetic research could appreciably advance knowledge about the treatment of disease. A system of interoperable databases would allow clinical researchers to track more efficiently any finding back to its basic scientific roots; conversely, a research scientist might track forward to postulate from hypotheses through potential applications on the basis of innovative uses of existing data (NIH, 1999b). Similarly, linkages between genetic databases or clinical databases and environmental exposure databases will be essential for understanding and modifying gene-environment interactions (National Research Council, 2002).

Other Large-Scale and Trans-NIH Science Initiatives

As a result of the success of the HGP, there is considerable interest in developing other larger scale projects with broad potential benefits. One well established example in cancer research is the Cancer Genome Anatomy Project (CGAP) of NCI. The goal of the CGAP is to develop gene-expression profiles of normal, precancerous, and cancer cells, which could be used by many investigators to search for new methods of cancer detection, diagnosis, and treatment. In addition to the CGAP, the number of large-scale initiatives in genomics involving multiple institutes has grown. The successful initiation of many of them depended on the institutional leadership at the time combined with growing budgets, according to Francis Collins, director of the National Human Genome Research Institute. In his presentation to the Committee, Collins described other plans for large-scale, trans-NIH projects that include building libraries of small molecules and tools for screening; longitudinal cohort studies to connect genotype, phenotype, and environmental risks; highly annotated databases of gene and protein structures and function; development of a computational model of the cell; and large-scale efforts in imaging and other population-based studies.

Recently, 18 institutes co-funded a bioengineering nanotechnology initiative, 12 co-funded initiatives in structural biology of membrane proteins, and 16 institutes and centers supported an effort in methods and measurement in the behavioral and social sciences.

The examples cited above indicate that there is some flexibility in NIH's administrative and priority-setting procedures to respond to new developments and allow for the initiation of large-scale research endeavors. However, recent funding patterns indicate that the institutes with the largest budgets, such as NCI, the National Institute of General Medical Sciences (NIGMS), and the National Heart, Lung, and Blood Institute, are more likely to initiate and support large-scale research projects. Smaller institutes do not have enough funds or flexibility in their budgets to begin such projects although they often leverage their resources through a larger institute's investment. It is not clear to what extent these projects are true collaborations in the sense that the participating institutes identify a challenge or an opportunity, work together toward developing a project, co-fund investigators and/or institutions, and manage and oversee the ongoing work. Thus, "multi-institute funding" should be distinguished from "trans-NIH initiatives," with the latter referring to activities that involve more than one institute in planning and implementation from start to finish.

Unanticipated fluctuations in annual congressional allocations and the appropriations process (which provides separate budgets for each IC) make strategic planning for new long-range, large-scale, or trans-NIH projects more difficult. In years in which the budget remains flat, new projects, especially large-scale new projects, are especially difficult to initiate. Moreover, because large-scale science is costly, it has the potential to reduce the funding available for the critical, but smaller, investigator-initiated projects. It is a bit more complicated for small research groups to initiate larger-scale projects because of the requirement that applicants for RO1 grants >$500,000 per year in direct costs obtain institute or center agreement at least six weeks prior to the anticipated submissions deadline before they can apply.[7] Thus, these requests require special budgetary and program planning in addition to scientific merit and budget justification. Applications submitted in response to NIH Program Announcements or Requests for Applications (RFAs), which include their own specific budgetary limits, are not subject to the same limits.

In addition to cost considerations, NIH management told the committee that true collaborations across institutes and centers can be made more difficult for a number of administrative reasons, such as: lack of clear support from leadership about the importance of such work; insufficient rewards for work conducted beyond the purview of an institute's specific mission; placement of "available" staff on such projects rather than individuals with the most appropriate skills or background; and insufficient financial resources and office space dedicated to get the work done.

NEW RESOURCE REQUIREMENTS: PATIENT DATABASES AND SPECIMEN BANKS

Other trends in biomedical science are influencing the importance of some kinds of data. For example, collections of archived patient information—including clinical data, family history, and risk factors—and such human biological materials as tissue, blood, urine, and DNA samples are essential for studying the biology, etiology, and epidemiology of diseases, especially if the diseases are linked. Such data can also be used to examine the long-term effects of medical interventions.

In 1999, the National Bioethics Advisory Commission estimated that more than 282 million specimens of human biological materials were stored in the United States and that they were accumulating at a rate of more than 20 million cases per year (NBAC, 1999). Maintenance, cataloging, and storage of these specimen banks and related data in a format that is widely accessible to the research community would require a long-term investment. Ensuring the quality and usefulness of specimen banks after the project-based funding ends is an unresolved issue now managed on a case-by-case basis.

The capacity to link medical records of individuals with family histories and disease phenotypes is an important point of departure for genetic analysis. Investigators at centers that have developed the capability and permission to search their patient database for informative patients and families will be well positioned to compete for the increasing proportion of federal and industrial research resources that will be devoted to genetic research, especially if non-genetic variables can be measured and linked (Silverstein, 2001; Omenn, 2000). Electronic medical records could make the work of specialists in one discipline widely accessible to specialists in many disciplines. If appropriate protocols can be developed, these records could

---

[7]NIH Notice for Acceptance for review of unsolicited applications that request more than $500,000 in direct costs, Effective June 1, 1998; see http://grants.nih.gov/grants/guide/notice-files/not98-030.html.

be used to integrate the work of clinicians with that of researchers and administrators, and could permit better and more rapid assessments of the health of the public in general and of individual patients in particular (Silverstein, 2001). It is important to note, however, that such electronic medical records would be available only in carefully reviewed and controlled circumstances under the federal Health Insurance Portability and Accountability Act and provisions of the Common Rule (45 CFR 46).

Electronically accessible medical records also could be used to track the health of the public in real time, for example, vaccine use or occurrence of hypertension, bacterial and viral pneumonias, cardiac arrhythmias, and sexually transmitted diseases. This would require substantial new federal money for equipment, personnel, and infrastructure and the expertise and resources of agencies other than NIH (Silverstein, 2001). In addition, the widespread use of the records raises a whole set of new ethical issues concerning privacy and confidentiality that must be adequately addressed if the public is to maintain its support for biomedical research. Nonclinical database links will be essential to address environmental, dietary, and behavioral interactions with genetic predispositions (Omenn 2000).

One issue that is common to all large-scale projects that generate research tools or databases is accessibility. Concerns are often raised regarding intellectual property rights, open communication among researchers, public dissemination of data and assuring protection of privacy and confidentiality. Explicit understanding must be negotiated and must be included in informed consent documents.

THE GROWING NEED FOR INTERDISCIPLINARY RESEARCH

Many of the projects described above are interdisciplinary. However, smaller-scale studies in the biological and biomedical sciences are also requiring more organized collaboration among disciplines. For example, data assessment, technology development, and a deeper understanding of science increasingly necessitate the involvement of non-biologists, such as engineers, physicists, and computer scientists. Recognition of the value of interdisciplinary research is not new. Indeed, the history of medicine demonstrates that many important advances have come from an interdisciplinary approach, for example, laser surgery involved ophthalmologists, anatomists, and physicists; and gene discovery, such as the cloning of the gene associated with Huntington disease, required the input of epidemiologists, neurologists, psychologists, sociologists, and geneticists. In fact, some of the newer fields in science are hybrid or trans-disciplinary efforts, such as bioinformatics, neuroscience, and health services research. The HGP has relied on the combined expertise of biologists, chemists, computer scientists, mathematicians, and engineers. In the behavioral sciences, psychologists increasingly use artificial intelligence, brain imaging, and molecular biology to map behaviors (Institute of Medicine, 2000). And psychiatric researchers long ago turned to epidemiologists and geneticists for help in identifying risk factors.

What is changing is the recognition that the need for interdisciplinary research is likely to grow. Some of the most persistent and chronic causes of disease, disability, and death are proving to be vexingly complex. Elaborate and sometimes subtle relationships among genes, environment, behavior, and disease and treatment interventions underlie HIV/AIDS, heart disease, autoimmune diseases, cancers, and substance abuse. Those conditions rarely lend themselves to the model of the single investigator working in isolation in their own discipline.

Most scientists would agree that the collective framing of research questions often leads to better answers. At the very least, most scientists are recognizing that the variables of interest and the tools of other disciplines might be useful in their own work. However, the organization of science and research administration, in academia and funding agencies, often presents challenges to interdisciplinary work. In 2000, an Institute of Medicine committee examining the need to foster interdisciplinary science in the brain, behavioral, and clinical sciences wrote that "long-held biases, beliefs, educational practices, and research funding mechanisms have created a system in which it is easier to conduct unidisciplinary than multidisciplinary work" (Institute of Medicine, 2000). The committee concluded that the creation of environments in which interdisciplinary research and training occur will probably require many changes and multiple integrated approaches. Creating a new breed of interdisciplinary scientists requires rethinking of the training process, including redesigning research training programs and funding mechanisms to support interdisciplinary training, research, and practice.

In 1999, NIGMS initiated a new funding mechanism referred to as glue grants, intended to provide the resources to bring together and retain scientists from multiple disciplines to focus on a research topic. In 2003, the Fogarty International Center announced a similar program. NIGMS's goal was to address problems that are beyond the reach of individual investigators who already held funded research grants related to a proposed topic of study. The RFA stated:

> Biomedical science has entered a new era where these collaborations are becoming critical to rapid progress. This is the result of several factors. First, not every laboratory has the breadth to pursue problems that increasingly must be solved through the application of a multitude of approaches. These include the involvement of fields such as physics, engineering, mathematics, and computer science that were previously considered peripheral to mainstream biomedical science. Second, the ability to attack large projects that involve considerable data collection and technology development require the collaboration of many groups and laboratories. Finally, large-scale, expensive technologies such as combinatorial chemistry, DNA chips, high throughput mass spectrometric analysis, etc., are not readily available to all laboratories that could benefit from their use. These technologies require specialized expertise, but could lend themselves to management by specialists who collaborate or offer services to others.

NIGMS originally conceived of the large-scale glue grants after consultations with leaders in the scientific community who emphasized the importance of confronting intractable biological problems with the expertise and input of large, multifaceted groups of scientists. Applicants are asked to consider what it would take to solve a problem if a team of investigators already funded were to coordinate and integrate their efforts and what approaches might be possible with the grant that cannot be achieved with just R01 support. Efforts to disseminate information are required, for example, meetings of participating investigators, newsletters, and Web sites. Materials produced as a result of glue grants are to be made as available to the wider community as is reasonable. One important objective of the glue grant program is to benefit a broad scientific community (beyond those named in the application).

TRENDS IN PUBLIC-PRIVATE SECTOR RESEARCH AND COLLABORATION

Changes in the financing, organization, and performance of R&D and technological innovation have altered how industry, research performers, and governments in the United States and elsewhere invest in research. According to the Pharmaceutical Research and Manufacturers of America (PhRMA), in 2001 member companies spent over $30 billion on research to develop new treatments for diseases—an estimated 17% of sales, a higher R&D-to-sales ratio than any other US industry. An additional $17 billion was spent on R&D by the biotechnology industry (Pharmaceutical Research and Manufacturers of America, 2001; Biotechnology Industry Organization, 2003).

Many initiatives—such as the SNPs Consortium, the mouse genome project, the structural genomics consortium, and the more general Small Business Innovation Research Program—have involved close collaborations between public funding agencies and private industry. Furthermore, numerous NIH institutes have started specific projects and grants that have been directed at enhancing public-private collaboration. Those experiments promise to deliver benefits to patient care. At the same time, they have raised important issues about intellectual property, ethical conduct of research, and conflict of interest that need to be addressed. The development of new products, processes, and services often entails gaining access to firm-specific intellectual property and capabilities.

> Firms and research performers have responded to these developments by outsourcing R&D and by forming collaborations and alliances to share R&D costs, spread market risk, and obtain access to needed information and know-how. Alliances, cross-licensing of intellectual property, mergers and acquisitions, and other tools have transformed industrial R&D and innovation. Universities have moved to increase funding links, technology transfer, and collaborative research activities with industry and government agencies. Government policies have supported these

developments through changes in antitrust regulations, intellectual property regimens, and initiatives in support of technology transfer and joint activities (NSF, 2002a).

In addition, numerous strategic research and technology alliances among a variety of institutions and enterprises, many involving international partners, have been created over the last two decades. Universities are important partners in these research joint ventures, participating in 16% of them from 1985 to 2000 (NSF, 2002a).

INCREASING INTERNATIONAL RESEARCH

The decline of global political blocs, expansion of convenient and inexpensive air travel, and advent of the Internet have facilitated scientific communication, contact, and collaboration. Data collected by NSF (2002a) show that the expansion of R&D efforts in many countries is taking place against a backdrop of growing international collaboration in the conduct of R&D. More R&D collaborations can be expected to develop with Internet-facilitated innovations such as virtual research laboratories and the simultaneous use of distributed virtual data banks by investigators around the globe.

In many countries, foreign sources of R&D funding have been increasing, and this underlines the growing internationalization of industry R&D efforts. In Canada and the United Kingdom, foreign funding has reached nearly 20% of total industrial R&D; it stands at nearly 10% for France, Italy, and the European Union as a whole. US firms are also investing in R&D conducted in other locations. R&D spending by US companies abroad reached $17 billion in 1999; it rose by 28% over a 3-year span. More than half that spending was in transportation equipment, chemicals (including pharmaceuticals), and computer and electronics products (NSF, 2002a).

A particularly notable international collaboration is the Human Proteome Organization (HUPO), which has launched international initiatives in characterization of proteins in plasma, liver, and brain and in underlying technologies, antibody resources, and bioinformatics (Hanash and Celis, 2002). NIH Director Zerhouni's Roadmap exercise identified proteomics as a leading enabling technology for new discoveries. NIH and FDA are closely involved with the not-for-profit HUPO, and several individual institutes have mounted their own proteomics workshops.

SUMMARY

Multiple trends are changing the nature and environment of biomedical research, including the persistent need for better approaches to clinical research, health services research, and evidence-based medicine; continuing concerns about health disparities; the looming threats of emerging infectious diseases and bioterrorism; the increased need for large-scale and trans-NIH projects that require longer-term strategic planning and commitments; the emergence of discovery-driven science and its attendant informatics and data requirements; the need to add new infrastructure elements to the nation's biomedical enterprise; the essential role of interdisciplinary research in many diseases; and expanding relationships between the public and private sector and between the United States and the rest of the world in research.

4

The Organizational Structure of the National Institutes of Health

A critical focus of the Committee's attention was the growing perception that the proliferation of the National Institutes of Health's (NIH's) institutes and centers (ICs) poses numerous problems for the agency, its leadership, and the overall effectiveness of its research and training portfolio in light of the new opportunities and challenges described in Chapter 3. As discussed briefly in Chapter 1, the Committee deliberated extensively on a variety of proposed responses to the changing nature of the biomedical frontier. Some observers have suggested maintaining the current array of ICs but grouping them in some way into "clusters," each of which would report to a deputy director, who in turn reports to the NIH director. That arrangement would maintain the existence of individual ICs and might encourage strategic planning within each cluster while reducing the number of subordinates with whom the NIH director must negotiate on strategy and direction. But the creation of a new management layer between the NIH director and the individual IC directors would, in effect, make the ICs divisions of larger organizations and might decrease the status, independence, and attractiveness of IC directorships and compromise the potential of the NIH director to provide appropriate strategic leadership.

Others, such as Varmus (2001), have suggested consolidating all existing institutes into five or six larger institutes of about equal size, whose leaders would report to the NIH director. Such a solution might well simplify some aspects of NIH management and some have suggested it might improve the overall effectiveness of the research portfolio. But it could also risk losing the support of many of the congressional, health advocacy, and public coalitions that have contributed so much to NIH's success. As noted in Chapter 1, the Committee believes that the development of NIH's current organizational structure has been a useful response to a set of complicated scientific and political influences. The Committee does not find the conceptual or practical case for a wholesale reorganization sufficiently compelling to outweigh its potential adverse consequences or risks. Rather, as laid out in this and subsequent chapters, the Committee makes recommendations for achieving many of the goals identified by proponents of major restructuring (more authority for the NIH director, increased responsiveness, greater flexibility, and more opportunity for coordination) primarily by other means.

The Committee is aware that many previous reports have recommended the adoption of a presumption against the continual addition of units to NIH. For example, the Special Committee on Medical Research, chaired by Cyril Norman Hugh Long in 1955 (NSF, 1955), concluded in its report that the seven institutes then in NIH were sufficient. Similarly, the President's Biomedical Research Panel stated in 1976 (Department of Health, Education, and Welfare, 1976), when there were 11 institutes, that "the creation of additional Institutes is not likely to make the NIH more effective; it might well make it less so. Therefore, if new programs are to be established, or existing programs strengthened, this should be accomplished through the present Institutes rather than through the creation of new ones." In the same year, the report of a Congressional panel chaired by Representative Paul Rogers (US House of Representatives, 1976) noted that the "categorical" structure of the institutes was a key to the success of NIH because it had given the public, Congress, and the administration a way to understand and identify with the mission of each institute. The Rogers report also noted, however, that NIH was facing pressure for too much categorization from advocacy interests not represented by name in the institute structure; "with eleven institutes, the problem of fragmentation becomes very real."

In 1984, an Institute of Medicine (IOM) committee chaired by James Ebert concluded that the current organizational structure of NIH was appropriate and effective (IOM, 1984). No new institutes had been created since 1974, but in the intervening decade, three institutes—the National Cancer Institute (NCI), the National Heart, Lung, and Blood Institute (NHLBI), and the National Institute for Arthritis, Diabetes, and Digestive and Kidney Diseases (NIADDK)—had been elevated to "bureaus," giving their directors more authority and the flexibility to create separate divisions to house major subunits of these institutes (NIH, 1976).[1] These changes were to accommodate health advocates' concerns, but pressures from

---

[1] As a result of the War on Cancer Act of 1971, NCI was elevated to a bureau with a greatly expanded budget and special authorities. NHLBI also became a bureau after the National Heart, Blood Vessel, Lung, and Blood Act of 1972 expanded its programs and budget; Congress added blood to the name of the institute in 1976. The NIADDK was raised to the bureau level in 1982, and separate divisions for diabetes, arthritis, digestive diseases, and kidney diseases were established. This was to respond to a report by the National Commission on Arthritis and Related Musculoskeletal Diseases that found the combination of topics under this institute's umbrella "incongruous." The bureau title has since been done away with (Cohen, 1993). See McGeary and Smith, 2002, for additional details.

outside groups were once again building for a separate institute for arthritis and a new institute for nursing. The 1984 IOM committee argued that "NIH is now at a stage where there should be a presumption against additions at the institute level because such changes (1) fragment the scientific effort and diminish effective communication with key scientists in other institutes, (2) add to the burden and difficulty of effective program coordination by the NIH Director and his top staff, and (3) add to administrative costs without ensuring increased appropriations." Because there might be circumstances in which organizational change would be necessary and it would be important to recognize such circumstances, the 1984 committee recommended that there be a formal process to assess proposed major organizational changes in NIH, and it articulated five criteria for evaluating organizational proposals:

1. "The activity of a new institute or other organizational entity must be compatible with the research and research-training mission of NIH. If a major emphasis of the proposed new entity is in regulation, the delivery of services, or other non-research activities, it is not appropriate for incorporation in NIH.
2. "It must be demonstrable that the research area of a new institute or other major organizational entity is not already receiving adequate or appropriate attention.
3. "There must be reasonable prospects for scientific growth in a research area to justify the investment in a new institute or other major organizational entity.
4. "There must be reasonable prospects of sufficient funding for a new institute or other major organizational entity.
5. "A proposed change in the NIH organizational structure should, on balance, improve communication, management, priority setting, and accountability."

Thus, the present Committee is hardly the first to consider these problems and deliberate over potential solutions. The Committee notes, however, that little changed as a result of past studies. The trend toward proliferation of units in NIH has continued to the present in the absence of an accepted process such as that suggested in the 1984 report.

NIH's continuing outstanding success has been due largely to its ability to adapt its programs and structure to meet the ever-changing needs and challenges posed by science, medicine, and public health. As already noted, the Committee carefully considered in multiple meetings major structural changes in NIH, including possible revisions in the number and reporting lines of ICs to the director, and concluded that a wholesale consolidation of NIH's ICs into a much smaller number of units is likely to generate more disadvantages than advantages. Nevertheless the Committee believes that a thoughtful process should be in place to respond to restructuring concerns as they arise to enable NIH to modify its structure as the situation warrants and NIH's continuing vitality demands. Because NIH is a public institution, the American public has a stake in its success and should be welcomed into decisions about its continued vitality and growth. A broad array of people and interests should be able to engage in thoughtful and balanced discussions about changes in NIH's institutional structure to address present and emerging issues even more effectively.

In line with these views, the Committee believes many changes in NIH's organizational structure and practices other than the number of ICs could potentially improve its effectiveness and help it to secure its continuing role in biomedical research. The Committee presents its recommendations on them in Chapters 5 and 6. The remainder of this chapter focuses specifically on issues surrounding the number of units (institutes, centers, and offices) in NIH and on the need to establish a more systematic process to address future needs for adding, consolidating, or dissolving structural units in response to changing scientific, health, or societal pressures.

PROCESS FOR CREATING NEW UNITS OR DISSOLVING OR CONSOLIDATING EXISTING UNITS

The Committee believes that it would be useful for Congress to consider amending the authorizing legislation for NIH to require that certain steps (outlined below) be taken in considering the creation, dissolution, or consolidation of new institutes and centers.

> **Recommendation 2:** *Public Process for Proposed Changes in the Number of NIH Institutes or Centers*
> Either on receiving a congressional request or at the discretion of the NIH director in responding to considerable, thoughtful, and sustained interest in changing the number of institutes or centers, the director should initiate a public process to evaluate scientific needs, opportunities, and consequences of the proposed change and the level of public support for it. For a proposed addition, the likelihood of available resources to support it should also be assessed and the burden of proof should reside clearly with those seeking to add an organizational element.

To initiate the process, the director should consult with the Advisory Committee to the Director and should a consensus develop on the value of further exploration, the NIH director should appoint an ad hoc investigative committee, ensuring that the appropriate array of technical expertise to evaluate a particular proposal is present and that the committee has appropriate representation of the extramural scientific and voluntary health advocacy communities.

Examples of steps it would be appropriate for the investigative committee to take include

- Inviting input from the advocates of the proposed action.
- Gathering input and opinion from the IC directors and other scientific leaders of NIH on the need for the proposed action.
- Soliciting the views of the Council of Public Representatives and other NIH advisory bodies.
- Holding a technical forum to be attended by the scientific community to address the scientific needs and opportunities related to the proposed action and the consequences of creating, dissolving, or consolidating one or more organizational units.
- Holding a public forum to gather the views of voluntary health advocacy organizations and other stakeholders.
- Consulting interested members and committees of Congress.

After the information-gathering steps, the investigative committee should synthesize a set of recommendations and report them to the NIH director. The NIH director would then deliver the investigative committee's report with his or her recommendations to Congress, indicating any important disagreements with the investigative committee. Congress should allow the process to conclude before acting to create a new unit or to consolidate or dissolve an existing unit.

Despite the present Committee's conclusion that a large-scale restructuring of the ICs would not be wise now, no organization that is expected to remain effective should have to bear the burden of a frozen organizational structure, and not all of NIH's existing units are likely to continue to have the same relevance or independence in the future. It is reasonable to suggest that the public, the scientific community, or the NIH director, in concert with internal and external advisers, should be able to suggest to Congress additions, subtractions, or mergers of units at appropriate times.

OPPORTUNITIES FOR MERGERS

After much consideration, the Committee came to the conclusion that a few ICs have overlapping missions and substantive foci and would work more effectively together than apart. The Committee suggests initiation of two careful studies to evaluate potential mergers. Those studies, however, would require time for detailed, open, and public evaluation of the issues as outlined in the process described above.

Two particular options were raised during Committee discussions as candidates for merging: the National Institute on Drug Abuse (NIDA) and the National Institute on Alcohol Abuse and Alcoholism (NIAAA); and the National Institute of General Medical Sciences (NIGMS) and the National Human Genome Research Institute (NHGRI). There are undoubtedly other mergers, additions, or closures that might be studied. The two suggested here are by no means an exhaustive list. The Committee, however, did not have the time or opportunity to review the merits of all such proposals to the extent that they deserve, which would include a thorough examination of the research and training programs of each institute under consideration. Indeed, the Committee favors these mergers, but believes that such changes should benefit from use of the process outlined above.

A Proposed Merger of NIAAA and NIDA

NIAAA and NIDA were originally parts of the National Institute of Mental Health (NIMH). NIAAA was established by congressional action as an organizational component of NIMH in 1970. In 1974, NIAAA, NIDA, and NIMH were made autonomous institutes under the newly created Alcohol, Drug Abuse, and Mental Health Administration (ADAMHA). With the dissolution of ADAMHA in 1992, NIMH, NIDA, and NIAAA were all transferred to NIH.

Over the years, there has been recurring interest in why the two institutes that focus on substance abuse and addiction are separate. As chair of the House Labor, Health and Human Services, and Education Appropriations Subcommittee, Representative John Porter asked the IC directors at every annual appropriation hearing why the two institutes had not been merged (Leshner, personal communication). More recently, questions have been raised in the Senate about the wisdom of keeping them separate,[2] and a National Academies study on the issue was strongly recommended in report language. To date, however, the method and implications of combining them have not been carefully investigated.

The arguments for combining the two ICs stem from overlap in their missions and substantive foci. The acting director of NIDA and the director of NIAAA noted the strong association between the use of tobacco and illicit drugs and the abuse of alcohol in a recent editorial in the *Journal of the American Medical Association* (Hanson and Li, 2003). Similar biological and social risk factors underlie vulnerability to all of these substances, and there are thought to be overlapping mechanisms in how these substances influence the brain. In addition, prevention and treatment approaches that are fundamentally similar for abuse of alcohol and other substances make it desirable from a public health perspective to address all substances of abuse when opportunities arise (Graham and Schultz, 1998).

Having two separate ICs focused on addictions has resulted in the emergence of two somewhat separate scientific communities, although some investigators receive support from both institutes. The existence of two scientific societies—the College on Problems of Drug Dependence and the Research Society on Alcoholism—and the fact that they have not convened scientific meetings together in the last 20 years provide dramatic evidence of segregation. Few studies investigate alcohol and other substances of abuse at the same time, even though few drug addicts abuse only one

---

[2]During the 107TH Congress, S. 304, the Drug Abuse Education, Prevention, and Treatment Act of 2001, as reported by the Senate Judiciary Committee on November 29, 2001, contained a provision that called for a study of a merger of NIDA and NIAAA by the National Academies. Although the bill was enacted as PL 107-273 in November 2002, the provision relating to the study was no longer included.

substance. And the exclusive focus of the two institutes on specific substances has meant that some addictions, e.g., gambling and food addictions, have received virtually no scientific attention.

Arguments against merger appear to be primarily nonscientific; for example, the alcohol industry might strongly and successfully oppose such a merger to avoid being associated, even indirectly, with considerations of illegal drugs. In the Committee's view, substantive arguments against merger are not convincing. One suggests that alcohol requires a separate institute because it is unique in affecting every cell in the body; but other abused drugs studied by NIDA, such as inhalants, also affect all cells. Another argument is that alcohol is unique among abused substances in being legal, at least for adults, and thus everything surrounding the drug is unique. On the other hand, NIDA supports a large amount of research on nicotine addiction, and smoking is also legal for adults. A merger of NIAAA and NIDA would seem to offer many advantages, scientifically and with respect to improved health, and should be studied carefully. The broader scientific relationships and physical location of these two institutes with other neurosciences institutes (especially NIMH and the National Institute of Neurological Diseases and Stroke) should also be considered.

A Proposed Merger of NHGRI and NIGMS

NHGRI was born out of NIGMS to give intense focus and impetus to the sequencing of the human genome. Established originally as a center and later elevated to institute status, NHGRI has done a superb job in leading the international effort to sequence and interpret the human genome. Its efforts have extended to the sequencing of the genomes of other organisms, whose comparative study has substantial benefits for health and other fields of research. Although the sequencing efforts have involved many other ICs, particularly NCI and NIGMS, as well as the Department of Energy and the biotechnology industry, NHGRI clearly has been the leader. Many other institutes have continued work on other aspects of fundamental genetics, including the genetics of various illnesses, and biomedical genetics has emerged as an overarching NIH high-priority field and a major venue for trans-NIH collaboration. Sequencing of the human genome was declared essentially complete on April 14, 2003, at the 50th anniversary celebration of the publication of the Watson and Crick paper on the double-helix structure of DNA. Biomedical researchers are building on the information to increase understanding of the functions of genes and the proteins they generate. Genetic medicine, genomics, and proteomics are among the core biomedical disciplines for the 21st century.

The Committee considered whether there is still a compelling need for a separate genome research institute. NHGRI's initial charge has been successfully accomplished, and having a continuing discrete focal point for human genomics might be useful for maintaining momentum in the field. However, it can be argued that NHGRI no longer has an essential separate mission. Many of its activities could easily be integrated into other ICs that have advanced their research as a result of the Human Genome Project and are integrating its findings into their missions.

Among the other institutes, NIGMS has core or primary responsibility for basic biomedical research. It can be argued that the same is true for genetics and that a core responsibility for NHGRI's projects should therefore be incorporated (actually, reincorporated) into NIGMS. In recent years, NIGMS has moved decisively into larger-scale transdisciplinary research, including glue grants (see chapter 3) and other mechanisms. On balance, the Committee believes that the completion of the human genome sequencing effort offers a good opportunity to study the possibility of combining the two institutes. Moreover, ending the life of NHGRI as a separate institute would, if determined to be appropriate, provide a dramatic precedent for declaring fulfillment of a well-defined mandate.

Consolidating Clinical Research Efforts

Because of extraordinarily persuasive arguments about exceptional needs made by a variety of groups in discussions with the Committee, a recommendation is made in this section to consolidate several clinical research components of the extramural and intramural program to transform the National Center for Research Resources (NCRR) into a new entity, the National Center for Clinical Research and Research Resources (NCCRRR).

The importance of clinical research in translating the vast knowledge emanating from basic science efforts, such as the Human Genome Project, cannot be overstated. As the result of a wide spectrum of developments in the biomedical sciences, extensive research can now be done on the pathogenesis and pathophysiology of human disease. In addition, new developments in imaging provide novel approaches to understanding the health and disease states in humans. As described in Chapter 3, the challenge for clinical research is that most common diseases are complex, multi-etiologic disorders in which a multiplicity of genetic and other factors interact with each other. As a result, clinical research is faced with the complex challenge of identifying the resources, intellectual capital, and large cohorts of patients with appropriate phenotypes for studies. It will take a revitalized investment in clinical research, including many large-scale trials, to figure out how to tie together all the factors that contribute to particular diseases.

Clinical research has always been more of an interdisciplinary "team" effort than laboratory science, but it will increasingly require larger, multi-institute studies and a level of collaboration, sharing, and cooperation that sometimes seems at odds with the image of the lone scientist working in isolation. German pathologist Werner Kollath once lamented, "Much is known, but unfortunately in different heads." If clinical research is to fulfill the promise of our nation's prolonged investment in biomedical research, then a more concerted and better coordinated effort must be mounted that will make the most of all available research and training resources.

NIH already sponsors a substantial set of programs in clinical research and training through its extramural and intramural research programs. It has continued to expand efforts to support clinical research and training and attract physician-investigators, often with strong encouragement from Congress and academic leaders. For example, it has established and expanded a series of special training programs for clinical researchers collectively known as K awards. And recognizing that loans accumulated during college and medical school greatly burden young physicians and influence their choices of career paths, NIH has responded by creating competitive loan-repayment programs that offer up to $35,000 per year for 2 years to health professionals pursuing careers in various aspects of clinical research.

The 87 general clinical research centers (GCRCs)—managed by the National Center for Research Resources (NCRR)—constitute a national network of NIH-supported clinical research sites hosted at academic health centers and teaching hospitals. They provide settings for medical investigators to conduct safe, controlled, state-of-the-art patient studies with support by the vast infrastructure of academic health centers. They also provide a crucial setting and mentorship to attract medical students, residents, fellows, and junior faculty—and patients and volunteers—into clinical research.

In addition, each institute or center with a research program supports a broad array of clinical research through individual research grants, research centers, and collaborative group funding mechanisms. Most ICs also conduct a variety of clinical research through the intramural program. As in the growing number of jointly funded extramural research programs, ICs may cooperate in studies. Such cooperation is facilitated by the intramural program's Clinical Center on the Bethesda campus.

NIH spent $7.6 billion on clinical research in FY 2002, estimates it will spend $8.4 billion of its roughly $27 billion budget in FY 2003 and projects spending $8.7 billion in FY 2004. The figures are complicated, however, in that the 20 clinically active ICs accounted for their "clinical research" efforts quite differently. However the funding is counted, almost all NIH institutes maintain substantial clinical research programs. For example, NCI, NHLBI, NIDA, and the National Institute of Allergy and Infectious Diseases maintain extensive clinical-trial research networks. Many institutes award contracts to conduct specialized research and clinical trials of potential treatments. Some institutes, such as NCI, NIMH, and NIDA, also support extensive arrays of research centers that provide infrastructure support and specialized clinical research project support.

NIH Director Zerhouni's Roadmap for Re-Engineering the Clinical Research Enterprise (Jenkins, 2002b; Metheny, 2003) outlines three pressures on the clinical research enterprise:

- the rate of growth of health care needs and expenditures requires accelerated discoveries and clinical validation;
  - new clinical approaches will have to be more efficient than current ones; and
  - public support and participation in clinical research are essential.

Many initiatives to bolster, support, and improve clinical research and training are under way at NIH, including public trust initiatives, the development of clinical research informatics, and planning meetings. An NIH Steering Committee on Clinical Research Infrastructure has been charged with defining the scope and purpose of clinical research informatics and ensuring sufficient external consultation to build a work plan for use of information technology in clinical trials. The plan will include data standards, core elements, model systems, and practices.

Even in light of NIH's considerable support of clinical research, the Committee sees a critical lack of coordination and standardization across NIH in its clinical research programs that cause many opportunities for collaboration and data sharing across fields to be lost. Clinical research is an expensive undertaking, requiring costly infrastructure and extensive administrative support to comply with regulatory requirements and interact effectively and efficiently in the financial and recordkeeping framework of clinical medicine. In addition, clinical databases can be sizeable and support for the necessary informatics daunting. In 2003, members of the Institute of Medicine's Clinical Research Roundtable published an article (Sung et al., 2003) characterizing the current state of clinical research as "increasingly encumbered by high costs, slow results, lack of funding, regulatory burdens, fragmented infrastructure, incompatible databases, and a shortage of qualified investigators and willing participants." The challenging and expensive enterprise of clinical research requires mastery of a broad array of skills in clinical medical fields; the application of biostatistics to clinical trial design and analysis; adherence to the principles, precedents, and procedures of bioethics; the organization and oversight of complex projects; and the communication of complex ideas to potential trial participants and peers. Sung et al. described two kinds of translational blocks: from basic science to human studies and from clinical knowledge to clinical practice, health-care decisions, and population health. The length of training required, the expense and time involved, and the complex regulatory environment of clinical research have depleted the ranks of those willing to engage in clinical research, and many feel that this trend contributes to the inability to translate basic research findings into improved health.[3]

To ensure the success of the clinical research system, there must be a cadre of highly trained clinical investigators for several reasons: to discern the questions to be asked; to ensure that studies are conducted with the highest quality standards; and to ensure that there are trained clinical investigators in all medical specialties enrolling patients in trials. As basic science discoveries outstrip clinical capabilities to apply them, the lag in translating clinical research to practice will continue to lengthen. This can only be addressed by providing coordinated support for stable and rigorous academic training programs, recruiting physicians to become scientists or continue their professional development through mid-career research training,

---

[3] An Institute of Medicine committee is currently developing a report on the role of academic health centers in the 21st century. The committee's report is still in preparation.

and ensuring that funds are available for clinical research proposals that seek to address significant problems in the diagnosis and treatment of human disease. For these reasons, it is critical that NIH concentrate its efforts to make the most effective use of what is already a sizeable investment.

NIH, the Association of American Medical Colleges (AAMC et al., 1999), and Sung et al. (2003) have concluded that NIH could enhance the contribution of the biomedical research enterprise to improved health in the United States and globally in numerous ways, including

- Working to build public engagement and trust in clinical research by creating new partnerships.
- Developing with the Department of Health and Human Services' Office for Human Research Protections a national approach to standardizing and harmonizing regulations for protecting research subjects and improving standards of privacy protection.
- Supporting the development of integrated, interoperable data networks, medical record systems, and related research under a common national health information infrastructure with standards to facilitate collection and sharing of clinical research information.
- Facilitating establishment of national and international clinical research consortia to study, standardize, and share information on disease prevention, pathophysiology, diagnosis, therapies, and outcomes.
- Strengthening the GCRC network to include more shared resources for clinical investigators.
- Creating national databases (consistent with the Health Insurance Portability and Accountability Act) that link the phenotypes, genotypes, risk factors, and multigenerational family histories of large numbers of people.
- Increasing opportunities (and funding) for clinical research training for physicians, dentists, pharmacists, public-health workers, nurses, psychologists, laboratory technicians, dieticians, computer programmers, bioengineers, and others, including education-loan repayment programs.
- Forging intergovernmental collaborations with related programs in the Department of Health and Human Services, such as the Centers for Disease Control and Prevention (CDC) and the Agency for Healthcare Research and Quality (AHRQ), as well as essential programs in the Departments of Veterans Affairs, Defense, Labor, and Agriculture.

The perceptions that more needs to be done to translate basic research into useful health interventions and that NIH could do more to promote and facilitate clinical and other research relating to the more effective implementation of new findings often result in calls for the creation of some new entity, whether inside or outside NIH, focused specifically on clinical research. For example, in May 2003, Senator Joseph Lieberman proposed the creation of a privately funded $150 billion

American Center for Cures, with the goal of supporting the translation of basic research discoveries into medical applications (Hawana, 2003). In the same month, the presidents of the Association of American Universities (AAU), AAMC, and the National Association of State Universities and Land Grant Colleges (NASULGC) in a letter to NCRR regarding its strategic plan, emphasized the importance of continuing to revitalize the GCRCs as a way to eliminate barriers to research progress and enhance investigator access to resources and technologies (Cohen, et al., 2003). The authors proposed merging NCRR's GCRC program with the NIH Clinical Center to form a national system dedicated to translational research.

The Committee also believes that the goals outlined above could be pursued better if the intramural and extramural clinical research programs of NIH worked more closely and collaboratively and if optimal use were made of the Clinical Center and the GCRCs, which together account for about 7-8% of the NIH budget. NIH is the ideal convener and organizer of a national clinical research enterprise and should lead a new effort throughout the biomedical research community to create and coordinate a national infrastructure for clinical research.

The Committee believes that the time is ripe for NIH to develop and implement a series of NIH-wide strategic initiatives in clinical research that engage the energies and resources of all ICs and recommends that even greater efforts be made than just merging the activities of NCRR and the Clinical Center, as proposed by AAU, AAMC, and NASULGC. A concerted, proactive effort requires that someone in a leadership position—with the attention of the NIH director and the authority to assess and coordinate efforts across NIH—systematically and routinely evaluate NIH's clinical research programs *in toto*. Those strategic initiatives should be aimed at facilitating the widespread incorporation of new concepts and technologies in molecular genetics, cell biology, imaging, computational biology, and information sciences into clinical research practice. Such strategic initiatives will advance the missions of all ICs and revolutionize health research. By this means, NIH's strategic investments in clinical research can have a transforming effect on the practice of medicine and public health in the United States. To achieve the goals outlined above, a more coordinated and concerted effort is needed.

Recommendation 3: *Strengthen Clinical Research*
NIH should pursue a new organizational strategy to better integrate leadership, funding, and management of its clinical research enterprise. The strategy should build on, but not replace, existing organizational units and activities in the individual ICs' intramural and extramural research programs. It should also include partnerships with the nonprofit and private sectors. Specifically, the Committee recommends that several intramural and extramural programs be combined in a new entity to subsume and replace the National Center for Research Resources, to be called the National Center for Clinical Research and Research Resources (NCCRRR). In addition, a deputy director for clinical research should be appointed in the Office of the Director to serve as deputy director and head of the new entity.

The Committee is well aware that there is already an associate director for Clinical Research at NIH who oversees the intramural Clinical Center. The new position of deputy director that we describe would, however, take responsibility for all combined intramural and extramural programs in clinical research.

The Committee gave careful thought to how to create the recommended new entity for clinical research. The most appealing option was to transform the NCRR into the NCCRRR, retaining its responsibilities for the GCRCs and K award programs and adding to these the oversight of the Clinical Center and the integration and coordination of other clinical research conducted by the ICs. The current NCRR director position would be replaced with a new position of deputy director for clinical research. Because NCRR would cease to exist, its non-clinical research programs, which are important, would have to be relocated to other venues in NIH. An attractive aspect of this option is that it does not create an additional direct report to the NIH director.

The Committee also considered other approaches, for example, moving the GCRCs, K award programs, Clinical Center oversight, and overall clinical research coordination to an institute or center other than NCRR, for example, to NHLBI. Although this option potentially could put clinical research into the hands of an entity well qualified to manage it, it could also create a lack of acceptance on the part of other institutes that might defeat the intent to improve trans-NIH integration of clinical research. Another idea was to create an entirely new center that combines the GCRCs, K award programs, Clinical Center, and coordination of IC clinical research under the direction of a newly created position of deputy director for clinical research. A major disadvantage of this option is that it would increase the number of direct reports to the director, which the Committee felt was undesirable. This could be avoided if the remaining parts of NCRR were relocated, as above, and the center was dissolved as a distinct entity.

The Committee decided that the best option is to build the new NCCRRR on the NCRR, adding to its responsibility for the GCRCs and the K awards for training and career development the oversight of the Clinical Center and coordination of clinical activities for which other ICs are responsible. If staff responsible for these critical aspects of NIH's clinical research and training portfolio report to a central office, there would be greater opportunity to enhance data sharing among clinical investigators, clarify, solidify, and standardize relevant policies, and identify and pool resources for high-cost, essential core infrastructure needs. A central location would also provide a well-informed opportunity for strategic planning. NCCRRR should have an advisory committee similar to those of other ICs (see also Chapter 6) and every effort should be made to ensure that investigators working in all aspects of clinical research have access to the services and resources of NIH and that the research agenda is not dominated by larger institutes.

The Committee understands that there is a concern about the functions of NCRR that are not related to clinical research, such as its primate centers. Those activities of the existing NCRR that are not focused on clinical research but that are nonetheless essential to the overall research enterprise should be maintained as offices or branches in appropriate other locations within NIH. The Committee believes that it should be left up to the NIH director to evaluate what current NCRR functions should be retained in the new NCCRRR and which ones to position elsewhere.

Each institute or center would continue to fund its own clinical research projects, collaborative groups, and trainees (as now through funding transfers to NCRR) and its use of the Clinical Center. Although planning at the Clinical Center emphasizes flexible cross-IC intramural use of the facility, it is envisioned that the new entity would assume a much stronger leadership role for the entire intramural and extramural NIH clinical research enterprise and work in close partnership with the academic community and the private sector. For example, the new Center could enhance and improve relations and ongoing discussions with clinical research organizations outside NIH, such as the Office for Human Research Protections, the Food and Drug Administration, CDC, AHRQ, and the pharmaceutical and biotechnology industries.

The goal would be to extend the resources and expertise of NIH's aggregate clinical research expertise more broadly, to more fully engage the clinical research community across the country and to develop standard tools and practices to promote clinical research. For example, two key areas in which the new Center could make enormous contributions are in information technology and clinical bioinformatics. Given the great expense of clinical trials, any increased productivity achieved through automation will have a substantial impact on the number of trials that can be successfully completed and on the speed of knowledge accumulation. Another important role could be in developing, through an inclusive process with the extramural community, the area of ethical conduct of clinical research and the setting of consistent national ethical standards for NIH grantees conducting clinical research.

The Committee believes that the importance of both intramural and extramural clinical research to all the ICs requires the full time and attention of one individual and his or her office within OD. Although the current and previous NIH directors have all strongly supported clinical research, it is just one of many missions that NIH must fulfill and thus has not received the full attention warranted, with efforts at promoting clinical research too ad hoc, too sporadic, and too subject to changes in NIH leadership. By consolidating many existing efforts into one organizational unit, clinical research would achieve maximal visibility and coordination.

SUMMARY

The Committee's conclusion was that, at the current time, a wholesale consolidation of NIH's ICs into a much smaller number of units would generate more disadvantages than advantages; however, a process to consider changing circumstances and suggestions for structural change as they arise is needed. The Committee believes that Congress should consider amending the authorizing legislation for NIH to require that either on receiving a congressional request or at the NIH director's discretion in responding to public requests for a structural change, the director should initiate a public process to evaluate the scientific, medical, financial, and public costs of the proposed change.

Some ICs have overlapping missions and substantive foci and would work together more effectively than apart, and the Committee recommends the immediate initiation of two careful studies using the recommended process to evaluate these mergers. In addition, the Committee recommends the merger of extramural and intramural functions related to clinical research.

5

Enhancing NIH's Ability to Respond to New Challenges

The highly decentralized organizational structure of the National Institutes of Health (NIH) has come about through a complex process of evolution over a long period marked by substantial increases in resources and extraordinary discoveries on the biomedical frontier. The evolutionary process involved numerous events and responses to pressures from a wide variety of interested constituencies that resulted in the creation of many largely independent organizational units. The governance of NIH has been profoundly influenced by that evolution. For example, Congress has created most additional units with their own budgets and decision- making authorities, which constrains the ability of the NIH director to influence the decisions and choices made by individual institutes and centers and makes the scientific leadership and management of NIH as a whole extremely challenging.

The Committee's view of those complexities was governed by the desire to be of practical assistance to all those who wish NIH to continue as an effective, indeed outstanding, organization, and it proceeded on the premise that its task included assessing the organizational configuration of NIH and the key processes and authorities that play roles in NIH-wide decision-making. Although the borders between structure, mission, and priorities are not well defined, the Committee tried not to take too expansive a view of its responsibilities.

On the one hand, a highly decentralized organization may be generally appropriate for a research organization because research and creativity often prosper through a bottom-up approach that encourages the flow of ideas from the widely dispersed scientific community and does not impede the role of individual investigators in choosing productive avenues of research. On the other hand, when there is a need for NIH to respond to important new health concerns or scientific opportunities—especially when inter-institute or "trans-NIH" initiatives are needed—the NIH director's authority to mobilize the needed resources is limited. There is no formal mandate for NIH to identify, plan, and implement cross-cutting strategic initiatives. In fact, the Committee has come to believe that NIH's current structure, governance, and management mechanisms have become barriers to its effectiveness in using its resources most efficiently to foster progress in large- and small-scale scientific endeavors that directly affect human health and that a more diverse set of mixed strategies for supporting research is essential.

As discussed in previous chapters, most of what NIH does should continue to operate as usual through activities and decision structures of the institutes and centers and the peer review system. Indeed, the Committee concluded that the existing NIH structure is fundamentally healthy and should continue to pay large dividends in scientific progress and meeting the nation's health needs. However, organizational changes should be made to increase NIH's effectiveness, improve its ability to respond to new scientific needs and opportunities, and thereby enhance its vitality. In this chapter, the Committee focuses on: planning and implementation of trans-NIH initiatives, which require more authority and resources for the director; development of a new mechanism to address high-risk research; and improvement in the NIH intramural research program's ability to move quickly and flexibly to meet urgent new needs and to work more collaboratively with the extramural research community.

THE AUTHORITIES OF THE DIRECTOR AND TRANS-NIH INITIATIVES

Despite the enormous success of NIH, and in part because of that success, the changing world of biomedical science and the stewardship of this great enterprise require increased attention to a number of critical scientific and health issues that no institute or center can address alone. In particular, as described in Chapter 3, over the last decade or more there has been growing recognition of the importance of both large- and small-scale interdisciplinary science, of the importance of strategic trans-institute initiatives, and of the increasing dependence of biomedical researchers on a broad array of new infrastructure investments. NIH has responded to those forces by, for example, sponsoring and successfully carrying out a number of large-scale interdisciplinary projects, such as cancer research and the Human Genome Project. Moreover, it has become increasingly clear that there is a high payoff potential for carefully selected large- and small-scale strategic projects that require the participation of numerous organizations working in partnership. Well-planned, broad-based, trans-NIH programs will be necessary to meet most effectively scientific or public health needs or to complete a task, with the assumption that at some point particular programs will have met their intent and cease to exist in any formal way. Although NIH has been successful in putting together some initiatives in which more than one institute co-funds a research program of mutual interest, it has not been as successful in jointly planned and implemented efforts across institutes. In this respect, the decentralized, federated structure and governance patterns of NIH are a disadvantage. Furthermore, there is no formal mandate for NIH to identify, plan, and implement such cross-cutting strategic initiatives.

In particular, the Committee believes that the difficulties encountered in initiating trans-NIH initiatives have been one reason why in the past some groups have called for new free-standing organizational units, which in turn has led to the proliferation witnessed over the past few decades. What might have been perceived as a lack of responsiveness on the part of NIH in some cases might have been more related to its inability to mount a sufficient response within the existing organizational framework.

The Committee suggests changes in the Office of the Director (OD) to improve the agency's agility and ability to respond to emerging scientific and health needs. These alterations would provide new mechanisms for selecting and planning strategic initiatives and would also give NIH an additional set of strategies for managing science—an approach the Committee concludes is not only appropriate, but also desirable.

The Authorities of the Director

The roles of the NIH director are to provide leadership and direction to the NIH research enterprise and to coordinate and direct important initiatives that cut across the agency. The OD is responsible for the development and management of policy for intramural and extramural research and training, the review of program quality and effectiveness, the coordination of selected NIH-wide program activities, and the administration of centralized support activities essential to the operations of the NIH. The director also oversees relationships between NIH and various other agencies in and outside the Department of Health and Human Services.

However, the NIH director has limited formal authority and OD lacks an adequate budget for its many roles. Institute and center (IC) directors have their own budgets, appropriated directly to them by Congress, which for the larger institutes, such as the National Cancer Institute (NCI) and the National Institute of Allergy and Infectious Diseases (NIAID), amount to several billion dollars. The NIH director has only a modest budget (see Table 5.1 in the section on the structure of the director's office, below) with a small discretionary fund ($10 million) and the authority to transfer up to 1% of the IC budgets to start new initiatives. An unanticipated decision to use that transfer authority during a fiscal year can prove highly problematic. The ICs, having typically committed their entire budgets, must cut funding for planned activities to accommodate an unexpected transfer. If a transfer is called for late in a fiscal year, the disruption to ongoing activities can be serious. Furthermore, even 1% of the budget might not be adequate for high-priority new initiatives. The reality is that the NIH director cannot mobilize important trans-NIH efforts to address new strategic goals because the authority for doing so is absent and he or she must rely largely on persuasion and goodwill to make even relatively modest changes.

The execution of current Director Zerhouni's "Roadmap" initiatives illustrates the problem well. Zerhouni has won much praise for his ambitious exercise to plan major new trans-NIH research projects, but their long-term future is by no means clear. Zerhouni has given notice that he intends to use the director's 1% transfer authority in FY 2004, and the President's budget request for FY 2004 contains an extra $35 million (0.1 percent of the NIH budget) for OD to implement the Roadmap. But no major new initiative is a 1-year effort, so sources for FY 2005 funding and beyond will be needed. Moreover, the committee believes that there should be, over time, a series of such initiatives. Ideally, FY 2004 initiatives would be adopted as part of the relevant ICs' regular research programs in FY 2005 and beyond, but the director has no authority to ensure that this happens.

Strategic Planning for Trans-NIH Initiatives

Although the Committee is not recommending a major structural reorganization of the NIH ICs, it concluded that to meet the scientific and health goals of the nation, NIH needs to mobilize coordinated funding from many institutes for high-priority time-limited initiatives that cut across individual institutes' purviews. The Committee believes that the best means to achieve that is through multiyear strategic planning that involves all ICs.

Scientific mechanisms, risk factors, and social and behavioral influences on health and disease cut across traditional disease categories. Many patients have multiple chronic conditions, so a patient-centered approach to health care and health promotion will sometimes require integration and synergy across ICs. For example, there have been recent calls for the establishment of an institute on obesity, which is a major public health concern. Because obesity is associated with diabetes, coronary artery disease, and arthritis, multiple NIH institutes could logically claim obesity as a critical component of their research portfolio. This is one of many potential topics that lend themselves to a strategic coordinated trans-NIH response in which multiple institutes could collaborate on a research plan that cuts across administrative structures in terms of planning, funding, and sharing and disseminating results. The Committee believes that a trans-NIH strategic initiative on obesity is a better mechanism to address this problem than the creation of a new institute. Proteomics, already cited by NIH Director Zerhouni as a critical enabling technology for discovery in the Roadmap, is another current example. Multiple institutes are independently holding workshops and considering or issuing Requests for Applications at a time when concerted trans-NIH work on the assessment of existing and emerging technology platforms and database formats utilizing reference specimens, could help to advance the whole field and guide NIH-supported studies. A trans-NIH initiative need not involve every IC and need not proceed indefinitely. But it would require dedicated funds, leadership, and scientific merit or it will not work.

NIH shared with the Committee evidence that the ICs are co-funding grants that account for about 20% of new awards, although the research topics of these awards have not been selected through NIH-wide strategic planning. It appeared to the Committee that, in many cases, these initiatives really involved only a few lead institutes that contributed the lion's share of the budgets. NIH managers told the Committee that these multi-institute programs are difficult to administer: they require sign-off by each institute involved, with each institute maintaining its own accounts and oversight. Thus, if five institutes are involved, there are five parallel administrative and oversight efforts in place.

Other efforts to improve cooperation and collaboration among institutes have met with limited success. For example, NIH intramural scientists have formed some 70 scientific interest groups across institutional boundaries. These groups are no doubt important forums for scientific exchange but they do not set priorities, plan programs, or expend research funds. A relatively new and path-breaking attempt at trans-NIH science is the consolidation of the intramural programs of the neuroscience-related institutes in the newly constructed Porter Center on the Bethesda campus. Other cooperative attempts, such as the NIH Pain Research Consortium—although well intended—have started and faltered over many years because funding generally has not been available and research programs are dependent on the willingness of individual institutes to fund specific projects (IOM, 2003b). The Committee was told in numerous interviews with NIH leadership that past efforts by the NIH director to "raise funds" from ICs to support trans-NIH initiatives have been viewed by the ICs as intrusions on their budgets. This is a direct consequence of the federalist structure of NIH and one this Committee would like to see reformed.

The Committee expects that many IC directors would see the expansion of such collaborations through planning and disbursement of research and training funds as an opportunity for leadership and leverage on topics important to them and their constituencies. To reiterate, the Committee is convinced that trans-NIH initiatives are a more direct and effective means to address emerging scientific and health improvement opportunities than is the creation of new centers or institutes.

The Committee concluded that the NIH director's authorities and resources must be increased to make it possible to achieve those goals. The Committee recommends that the director be given the responsibility and authority to develop and implement, with and through the ICs, a set of time-limited trans-NIH initiatives that are identified through a broad-based strategic planning process open to participation by all internal and external stakeholders and transparent to the public. Such a process should be conducted regularly, for example, every other year. The Committee envisions the process producing a sufficient breadth and diversity of initiatives to make it readily feasible for each institute and center, with the director, to identify one or more initiatives that are compatible with its own mission and goals in which to participate. In fact, the Committee is convinced that such a requirement from Congress is likely to stimulate ICs to propose and even lead trans-NIH initiatives. In any case, each institute and center should be required to reserve a substantial portion of its budget for such participation, starting initially at a few percent, but increasing over the next 4-5 years to 10% or more if initial efforts prove successful. The Committee believes that the initiatives will, over time, allow each of the institutes and centers to pursue its goals and interests more effectively. The Committee envisions the strategic initiatives selected through the planning process being temporary in the sense that their status as "new initiatives" will extend only through one or a few planning cycles, after which other initiatives will take their place. However, as the work involved in these initiatives is performed, the Committee expects that at least some elements of the work will spin off into new components in the portfolios of many of the ICs that become part of their regular research agendas. In addition, many activities covered by existing grants and programs are likely to be relevant to some strategic initiative topics, and could become part of IC participation in the trans-NIH initiatives if the NIH director's review confirms their appropriateness for inclusion. That is, an institute or center could include aspects of existing programs in its trans-NIH obligation with confirmation from the director that they are relevant and should be counted as part of the IC's participation.

The Committee identified several options for organizing and managing a trans-NIH budgeting process:

- Sufficient funds (for example, 5% of the NIH budget would be about $1.5 billion) could be appropriated to OD for the NIH director to make allocations to the participating ICs through the planning process.
- The target proportion of funds appropriated to each institute or center could be treated as though "in escrow" until the NIH director affirms that the unit has committed its expenditure for one or more of the identified trans-NIH initiatives of relevance to it.
- The use of the target proportion within each IC budget could be left to the IC and its director, with retrospective review by the NIH director and Congress. The annual performance review of the IC director would include attention to this element.

In the Committee's view, the second, or "escrow," option is preferred. The NIH director should have the authority to require the necessary funding commitments from the ICs for their participation in the initiatives chosen, but the committed funding should not be transferred either to the NIH director or to another IC. Rather it should be set aside to represent each unit's participation in furthering the chosen research initiatives. The initiatives should be carried out extramurally through multi-unit grant or contract programs, or as a combination of multi-unit extramural and participating unit intramural efforts.

The implementation of each of the initiatives should be overseen by special temporary task forces formed for this purpose with representation from each of the participating ICs. The commitment of the ICs should be reflected in the assignment of excellent staff to trans-NIH task forces on a full-time basis. As appropriate, NIH should also periodically sponsor scientific symposia to inform the relevant NIH constituencies and the director of progress on each trans-NIH strategic initiative.

Such a process would give NIH a capacity to respond to newly identified health needs in a coherent organization-wide manner. Together, the initiatives would have the effect of greatly expanding trans-NIH research and cooperation and breaking down barriers among IC research agendas. It might also make the NIH research enterprise more efficient and less apt to duplicate effort. Although OD would lead the process, its consensus-driven nature would incorporate the views of NIH's many internal and external constituencies and provide the potential to increase understanding and satisfaction of the external scientific and health advocacy communities.

Recommendation 4: *Enhance and Increase Trans-NIH Strategic Planning and Funding*

a. The director of NIH should be formally charged by Congress to lead a trans-NIH planning process to identify major cross-cutting issues and their associated research and training opportunities and to generate a small number of major multi-year, but time limited, research programs. The process should be conducted periodically—perhaps every 2 years—and should involve substantial input from the scientific community and the public.

b. The director of NIH should present the scientific rationale for trans-NIH budgeting to the relevant committees of Congress, including a proposed target for investment in trans-NIH initiatives across all institutes. For example, an average target of 5% of overall NIH funding in the first year, growing to 10% or more over 4-5 years, may be appropriate.

c. The appropriations committees should annually review budget justifications and testimony from the NIH director and from individual IC directors about the participation of each unit in the planned trans-NIH initiatives and the portion of their budgets so directed. Congress should include budget targets in the appropriations report language. The Committee recommends beginning with 5% of the overall NIH budget.

d. To ensure that each IC uses the target proportion of its budget for trans-NIH initiatives of its choosing, that proportion of the annual appropriation to each unit should be treated as "in escrow" until the NIH director affirms that the unit has committed to its expenditure for the identified trans-NIH initiatives.

e. The President should include in the budget request, and Congress should include in the NIH appropriation for OD, funds to support an appropriate number of additional full-time staff to conduct the trans-NIH planning process and "jump-start" the initiatives that emerge from this process.

Once again, the Committee believes that IC directors should view such planning as an opportunity for leadership and leverage on topics important to them and their constituencies and as a means for adapting their missions to new developments. Advocacy organizations, scientific societies, and NIH advisory bodies, including the Council of Public Representatives, likewise should see this process as an opportunity to gain synergies across the many interrelationships among diseases. If they do, the commitment to the trans-NIH task force should be reflected by the assignment of staff on a full-time basis, a career assignment viewed as a plum. The structure to accomplish the trans-NIH initiatives identified in the strategic process could take several forms depending on the size of the initiative, the number of institutes that need to be involved, and the likely time it will take to see the initiative to fruition.

The Committee recognizes that the prospects for putting new and significant trans-NIH objectives into practice will be affected by the growth of the NIH budget. If all existing programs continue to enjoy the highest priority there will likely be resistance in the early years of the initiative by institutes that claim difficulty in meeting their commitments while still offering some new grants. As a result the NIH director will have to exert superb and compelling leadership to withstand requests to release "escrowed" funds from trans-NIH projects. For these reasons, it is particularly critical that IC leadership comes to view participation in these initiatives as beneficial, and that Congress ask IC directors to report each year on the extent to which they are participating.

THE STRUCTURE OF THE OFFICE OF THE DIRECTOR

More than 40 unit heads report to the director—the directors of 27 ICs, the heads of 4 program offices and the heads of 12 staff offices in OD. Although the FY 2002 budget of $239 million for the OD may seem ample, the vast majority of this funding was earmarked for the support of a group of program offices and special programs, and that has been the case since 1993. (See Table 5.1.) The composition of the earmarked amount has changed regularly, however, as OD has been used as an incubator for offices and programs that were established and then spun off as centers or institutes or absorbed into existing institutes. For example, the Office of Alternative Medicine became the National Center for Complementary and Alternative Medicine in 1998, the Office of Research on Minority Health became the National Center on Minority Health and Health Disparities in 2000, and the Office of Bioengineering and Bioimaging became the core of the new imaging and bioengineering institute in 2000.

To carry out the responsibilities of managing, planning, and coordinating the programs of the 27 ICs, the NIH director is assisted by a number of staff units collectively called OD Operations. A series of staff offices are headed by associate

TABLE 5.1 Office of the Director Appropriations—FY 1993-FY 2003
(in thousands of dollars)

	1993	1994	1995	1996	1997	1998	1999	2000	2001	2002 (est'd)	2003 (req'd)
OD Operations	40,825	42,001	44,722	44,688	45,882	49,505	52,563	55,083	66,874	76,730	83,277
Director's Discretionary Fund	10,329	6,322	7,276	11,362	8,363	9,960	10,000	10,000	9,874	10,000	10,000
OAR	13,965	24,538	24,107	27,550	35,561	40,459	43,289	44,653	48,218	53,786	58,322
AREA Program	12,861	13,234	12,677	14,087	14,003	14,674	16,547	17,239	17,966		
Science Education	1,747	1,813	1,696	1,865	2,225	2,504	2,969	3,091	3,219	3,565	3,874
ORMH	9,037	9,794	8,923	8,920	8,825	9,839	10,741	11,367			
Minority Health Initiative	40,768	54,813	58,210	62,474	62,406	66,101	75,343	86,248			
ORWH	9,425	10,204	13,505	16,142	16,184	17,105	19,592	20,396	22,046	37,385	40,672
Loan Repayment Program			954	2,781	2,742	3,118	3,920	4,081	6,981	6,239	6,785
ORD			750	1,238	1,481	1,541	1,985	2,068	2,159	10,359	11,269
ODS				999	974	1,493	3,487	4,966	9,966	17,022	18,520
OBSSR			2,265	2,191	2,433	2,631	12,794	19,828	20,648	23,738	25,825
Foundation for the NIH					200	500	500	500	500		
OBB								200	1,970		
OAM	1,973	3,386	5,374	7,737	11,967						
LDRR	1,908	1,997	1,767	1,996	2,018						
Neurodegenerative Initiative					7,977						
Pediatric Initiative					4,976						
Women's Health Initiative	41,559	59,121	56,915	56,472							
Extramural Construction	4,949										
EARDA					1,500	1,500	1,905	1,984	2,067		
TOTAL	189,346	227,223	238,341	260,482	229,717	220,930	255,635	281,704	212,482	238,824	258,544

Source: For FY 1993-FY 2000, table provided by Office of the Budget, NIH; for FY 2001-FY 2003, table in FY 2003 NIH Congressional Justification Budget, Vol. V, p. OD-26 (DHHS, 2002), on-line at http://odeo.od.nih.gov/intra/budget/fy03odcjnarrativefinal.pdf. Figures for FY 2001, updated by NIH subsequent to submission of the FY 2003 budget, are used here.

directors. They include the Office of Science Policy, the Office of Budget, the Office of Communications and Public Liaison, the Office of Legislative Policy and Analysis, several components of the Office of Management—Financial Management, Human Resource Management, and Research Services—and several other units.

The FY 2002 budget for OD Operations was less than $80 million. Although the OD Operations offices assist the director in managing NIH, they are small and their budgets have not grown in proportion to NIH's research funding. The OD Operations budget increased by 88% from 1993 to 2002 compared with 125% for all of NIH. It amounts to 0.3% of the total NIH budget, down from 0.4% in 1993. Because of the tight budget for OD Operations, when unforeseen needs surface, as has happened recently with the development of stem cell research policies and harmonizing the rules for human subjects protection, OD is likely to have to "pass the hat" to the ICs to gather the additional resources needed. The Committee believes that the director should be given either a more adequate budget to support OD's management roles or greater discretionary authority to reprogram funding from earmarked components of the OD budget when necessary to meet emerging needs. Funding for OD Operations has not kept pace as NIH has expanded and has not grown in proportion to NIH's research budget; it is the Committee's view that it is inadequate for the effective management of the organization.

> Recommendation 5: *Strengthen the Office of the NIH Director*
> The Office of the Director should be given a more adequate budget to support its management roles or greater discretionary authority to reprogram funding from the earmarked components of its budget when necessary to meet unanticipated needs. In particular, if the director is given the responsibility and authority to conduct NIH-wide planning for trans-NIH initiatives, the director's budget will need to be amplified to take the costs of such planning into account.

In addition, the earmarking of funds by Congress for the establishment and continuation of programmatic offices in OD sometimes limits the director's flexibility and fluidity of resources, as well as his or her ability to effect change across the organization. It is difficult to ascertain whether the programmatic offices within OD have achieved their intended goals. Certainly, offices that move up and out to become centers or institutes reach the level of prominence desired by their advocates. But when the creation of an office in OD does not accomplish what the advocacy community desires, it increases the pressure for elevation of that office to a higher-level unit. The Committee believes that the process recommended in Chapter 4 for evaluating the merits of proposed additions to or subtractions from the list of ICs should also be applied to the creation of new offices in OD itself. The Committee is concerned that the creation of programmatic offices in OD could defeat the purpose of efforts to draw greater attention to important cross-cutting concerns because the creation of an issue-oriented office in OD tends to shift the responsibility for that issue to OD and away from the ICs, thereby reducing the attention that it might deserve. The time may be right to assess the effect that the programmatic offices in OD have had, including their role in the NIH director's policy and planning processes, whether the programs have clear goals, and whether there is a need to "sunset" an office once it achieves its goals.

> Recommendation 6: *Establish a Process for Creating New OD Offices and Programs*
> The public process recommended in Chapter 4 (Recommendation 2) for evaluating a proposal to create a new institute or center or to consolidate or dissolve institutes or centers should also be used for a proposal to create, consolidate, or dissolve offices in OD. The process should be used to evaluate the scientific needs, opportunities, and consequences of the proposed change, the likelihood of resources being available to support it, and public support for it.

FOSTERING HIGH-RISK, HIGH POTENTIAL PAYOFF RESEARCH

To increase investment in high-risk, high potential payoff research, the Committee also believes that there is a need for a "Director's Special Projects Program" external to the budgets of the ICs and funded as an OD line item. The goal of the program would be to fund the initiation of high-risk, innovative research projects. In a broad sense, the Committee imagines the program to be patterned after the Defense Advanced Research Projects Agency (DARPA), but with important differences.

The current peer-review mechanism for extramural investigator-initiated projects has served biomedical science well for many decades and will continue to serve the interests of science and health in the decades to come. NIH is justifiably proud of the peer review mechanism it has put in place and improved over the years, which allows detailed independent consideration of proposal quality and provides accountability for the use of funds. However, any system that focuses on accountability and high success rates in research outcomes may also be open to criticism for discriminating against novel, high-risk proposals that are not backed up with extensive preliminary data and whose outcomes are highly uncertain. The problem is that high-risk proposals, which may have the potential to produce quantum leaps in discovery, do not fare well in a review system that is driven toward conservatism by a desire to maximize results in the face of limited funding resources, large numbers of competing investigators, and considerations of accountability and equity. In addition, conservatism inevitably places a premium on investing in scientists who are known; thus there can be a bias against young investigators. The current steep decline in the growth rate of the NIH budget proposed in the President's FY 2004 budget may make it even less likely that high-risk proposals will be funded.

The DARPA approach specifically seeks high-risk research and expects failures—a marked difference from the NIH study sections or the consensus approach of committees. DARPA's mission is to develop imaginative and innovative ideas that have the potential for important defense-related technological impact. Such an impact is, however, by no means guaranteed. DARPA was developed specifically to foster research focused on high-risk, high potential payoff technology development. Typically, DARPA research establishes feasibility, and the results are handed off to other branches of the military services for development. The process has been successful: DARPA can claim credit for the foundational research that led to many noted and highly recognizable accomplishments, such as the Saturn rocket (1960s); the M-16 rifle (1970s); the Stealth fighter, global positioning system, and Arpanet/internet (1980s); the Predator unmanned aircraft (1990s); and the Global Hawk aircraft (2000s). Results of DARPA projects were also influential in the development of the National Science Foundation's (NSF's) nanotechnology and computer sciences programs (Betz, personal communication). It must be noted that much of the research funded by DARPA results in failure, which is the *expected* price of the quest for unusual breakthroughs.

Cook-Deegan (1996) provided examples of how real situations in the past might have been helped by the presence of a DARPA-like entity at NIH. In 1981, both NIH and NSF turned down a request from Leroy Hood and colleagues at Caltech for funding to automate DNA sequencing. The Caltech researchers subsequently obtained funding from the Weingart Institute instead, and by 1984 had made sufficient progress in prototype development to win NSF funding. Their method eventually became the dominant one on the market. In 1989, the National Center for Human Genome Research held a peer reviewed competition for large-scale DNA sequencing. It took about a year to develop and announce the competition and another year to review proposals and make funding decisions, but two years is a long time in a fast moving field. Ultimately the process rejected proposals from J. Craig Venter and Leroy Hood to do automated sequencing and selected a technology that was already a decade old. Hood's and Venter's subsequent successes in speeding up various sequencing efforts are well documented.

Cook-Deegan notes that many people assume that DARPA's approach is only suitable for engineering and technology development, but not pure science. "Experience suggests otherwise, however. Packet switching for electronic communication, computer time-sharing, integrated large-scale chip design, and networking were as conceptually 'basic' when DARPA was funding them as most molecular biology experiments are today." It is not difficult to identify research areas in today's biomedical science that might benefit from such an approach, for example, optics in neuroscience. Miller (2003) reported that in vitro studies of cultured neurons and brain tissue have built-in limitations for understanding how learning takes place in the brain. The "wish list" of neuroscientists includes finding a way to visualize individual neurons and track minute changes in the cells' structure and electrical activity; using two-photon microscopy to peer about half a millimeter into the brain to visualize the cortex and see into the unanesthetized brain; and finding a means to visualize deeper structures, such as the hippocampus. Fulfilling this wish list could bring about an optical revolution in neuroscience, but many of the needed techniques remain far off.

The Committee is aware that a number of alternative pathways might be used to establish a greater capability to support high risk research at NIH. NSF, for example, maintains a program of Small Grants for Exploratory Research (SGER) and allows its program officers to fund a limited number of small-scale, exploratory, and high-risk research projects at their own discretion subject only to internal NSF merit review. Such projects focus on preliminary work on untested and novel ideas, the application of new expertise or new approaches to "established" research topics, and work having extreme urgency with regard to availability of or access to data, facilities, or specialized equipment, including quick-response research on natural disasters and similar unanticipated events (NSF, 2002b). The SGERs are limited to $100,000. As Cook-Deegan (1996) points out, this is a good idea, but there is no reason to think that innovative projects will always be small. The Committee believes that a mechanism to promote high-risk research at NIH must allow for larger scale efforts to be effective. Another approach might be to experiment with the idea of a DARPA-like program with a pilot in only one or a few ICs. The Committee believes, however, that such an approach is likely to have limited success for two reasons. First, the establishment of such a program inside one or a few ICs is bound to limit its scope to the topical areas already in the ICs' portfolios, which could partly defeat its purpose. Second, locating such a program inside one or a few ICs would make it overly subject to their prevailing culture, which is already biased against high-risk research. (It should be noted that DARPA was created to report to a high-level Department of Defense official outside the research organizations of the military services to protect it from the hostility of those services, which sought to eliminate it. Augustine, personal communication, 2002.) The Committee believes that the proposed Director's Special Projects Program would have its best chance for success if it were located in OD and had a leader who reports to the NIH director.

The proposed Director's Special Projects Program at NIH would, like DARPA, be designed to foster the conduct of innovative, high-risk research. Research initially funded through the program that generates useful results would be handed off after 3-5 years for further development and funding through the standard NIH peer-review mechanisms of the ICs. If positive results were not generated after a reasonable period of time, as is anticipated for much of this type of research, the projects would be terminated. The Committee expects that there would be clear missions and finite life spans for these projects and that multidisciplinary teams of investigators would perform most of them.

The heart and soul of DARPA are its program managers, the scientists and engineers who initiate and oversee the research programs. They are responsible for developing program ideas and choosing contractors to perform the research, usually at universities or in industry. (DARPA has no intramural research program.) The program managers are not permitted to spend more than 4 years at the agency.

During their tenure, they have much autonomy in initiating programs and in choosing the investigators to be funded. DARPA reports to the Department of Defense's director for Defense Research and Engineering and operates in coordination with but independently of the military research and development establishment.

A cadre of talented program managers to select and manage the projects under the NIH Program could be drawn from academia, industry, and the ranks of NIH intramural scientists. Their most important feature would not be their previous affiliations, but rather that they are "idea people," capable of developing or recognizing unusual concepts and approaches to scientific problems. As at DARPA, the program managers would be appointed to strictly limited terms (such as 2-4 years) that are not renewable. The limitation on terms ensures that the programs are continually infused with fresh ideas and talent, which is thought to be a key reason that DARPA has been successful. The Committee believes that the NIH program managers should be able to accept ideas—either through unsolicited proposals or more directed responses to requests for applications or through peer review when appropriate—from the extramural and intramural scientific communities, as well as drawing on their own ideas. In addition, to allow for appropriate peer review, review panels specifically charged with selection of high-risk, high potential return projects could be constituted outside the standard peer review mechanisms to assist the program managers in selecting projects for funding.

The Committee believes that such a program will have its best chance to succeed if Congress provides new funding. The Committee suggests that a budget of $100 million for FY 2005 would be appropriate to initiate the program with a full-time program director and four to six program managers. Because it is likely that it will take 8-10 years for the program to reach full maturity, a commitment to keep it going at least this long should be made. The Committee envisions the program's budget increasing over the 8-10 years to as high as $1 billion per year.

> Recommendation 7: *Create a Director's Special Projects Program*
> A discrete program, the Director's Special Projects Program, should be established in OD to fund the initiation of high-risk, exceptionally innovative research projects offering high potential payoff. The program should have its own leader, who reports to the director of NIH, and a staff of short-term (2-4 years) program managers to manage identified projects with advice on program content from extramural panels. The program should be structured to permit rapid review and initiation of promising projects; if peer review is deemed appropriate, the program should use peer review panels created specifically for it and charged with selecting high-risk, high potential return projects. Congress should be prepared to provide new funding in the amount of $100 million, growing to as much as $1 billion per year for this endeavor, and commit to support it for at least 8-10 years so that a sufficient number of projects can reach fruition and a full assessment of program efforts can be made. A program review should be conducted during the fifth year to provide mid-course guidance.

Consistent with Recommendation 5 on sufficient funding for OD, this recommendation requires that the NIH director have the resources to hire first-rate scientists to help manage these increased responsibilities for developing programs.

THE INTRAMURAL RESEARCH PROGRAM

The performance of the NIH intramural research program (IRP) has been evaluated several times in the last 25 years by advisory groups in response to administrative and legislative mandates. The evaluations included a review of NIH by the President's Biomedical Research Panel (Department of Health, Education, and Welfare, 1976), an Institute of Medicine report (IOM, 1988), a report by the Task Force on the Intramural Research Program of the National Institutes of Health (NIH, 1992a), and the report of the External Advisory Committee on the Intramural Research Program (NIH, 1994). That might seem to be an excess of scrutiny. But one might equally wonder whether the repeated calls for review reflect a continuing concern about the quality of programs and performance and a lack of response to criticism and recommendations. The IRP has faced persistent difficulties, including problems with recruitment and retention of senior scientists, expansion of a postdoctoral training program of uncertain and uneven quality, cumbersome administrative requirements, inadequately funded congressional and administrative mandates, and deteriorating facilities, in particular in the Clinical Center.

Like the extramural program, the IRP has a fragmented federated structure. The IRP, with its $2.5 billion annual budget, comprises 19 separate intramural programs associated with the individual ICs. Just as each institute has a different legislative history and mandate from Congress, their IRPs vary widely in goals, scope, and size. Prior reviews have found this administrative structure to hinder unified or effective management of the IRP by the OD and to contribute to unevenness in quality, quality control, and productivity across NIH.

The IRP's proportion of the total budget has been reduced to only about 9 or 10% of the total NIH budget today and the IRP's budget growth has in recent years been deliberately slowed. Despite those reductions in the program, the question of what makes the IRP unique still recurs. In the past, the justification for the program was that it has distinctive input characteristics, including relatively long-term and stable funding of research programs, the availability of the Clinical Center's patient investigational facilities, few or no distractions from research for scientists, and a primarily retrospective, rather than prospective, review process for maintaining scientific quality.

For many years, the NIH campus was an exceptional training ground, especially for clinical investigators. Indeed, a large fraction of the senior leadership of the extramural biomedical research community received its training in the NIH IRP in the 1960s and 1970s. But the rapid growth in the NIH extramural program enabled biomedical research across the country to expand in size and scope, providing superb opportunities for training at academic facilities elsewhere.

The most recent of the IRP evaluations, by the External Advisory Committee (EAC) of the Director's Advisory Committee, also known as the Marks-Cassell committee, originated because of concerns expressed by Congress and others regarding the quality, appropriateness, size, and cost of the NIH IRP. In its many recommendations to the NIH director, the EAC concluded that the problems plaguing the IRP, unless addressed, "may destine it to a mediocre future." The committee identified many areas of concern:

- The review process for tenured scientists and scientific directors,
- The review process for appointment to tenure,
- Postdoctoral training,
- Administrative issues affecting recruitment and retention,
- NIH-private sector collaborations,
- The process for allocating funds between the extramural and intramural programs, and
- Renewal of the Clinical Center.

The EAC recommended that each institute be subjected to an individual review along lines proposed by the EAC.

In response to the EAC report, NIH prepared and implemented a plan to address the review process for tenured scientists, a tenure-track program, and changes in postdoctoral recruitment and training. In addition, progress has been made in removing some of the administrative impediments to research and in enhancing the attractiveness of employment in the IRP through changes in the pay scale and retirement options for senior investigators. Some ICs implemented the IC-level reviews recommended by the EAC.

The present Committee, given the time and resources available for it to complete its task, did not attempt to evaluate the quality of the IRP systematically. The Committee is, however, persuaded that the significant efforts of recent years to reinvigorate the IRP and respond to various advisory committee recommendations have met with considerable success and that there has been a promising trend toward improved overall quality in the IRP. The Committee applauds the efforts of the NIH deputy director for intramural research to improve the program overall. Nevertheless, the balkanization of the IRP persists because of its multiple institutional budgetary and programmatic lines, which reinforce the "stove-piping" and continue to make it difficult for the senior management of NIH to ensure that the IRP supports NIH's overall strategies and plans. The Committee therefore suggests that it would be useful to consider mechanisms to foster interactions among the IRPs of the individual ICs, such as large-scale reassignments of space to bring similar programs in individual institutes together to create synergies. It might also be useful to explore reducing the balkanization of the IRPs by clustering programs that share common themes, approaches, and tools, similar to the approach currently being taken to integrate the neurosciences in one building.

The Committee is convinced that the IRP should not merely be an internal extension of the extramural community, but rather should be doing distinctive research that the extramural research community cannot, or will not, undertake. The Marks-Cassell committee stated that "quality—not necessarily uniqueness, should be of the highest priority in determining support for the intramural research program." The present Committee does not fully agree with that statement, especially with its implementation, which typically has ignored uniqueness. Too little weight has been placed on the need for distinctive contributions by the IRP. Uniqueness and quality should both be essential justifications of the IRP, and it is not clear what distinguishes many of the current activities of the IRP from programs conducted by the extramural community.

Although evaluation of the quality of the clinical research protocols conducted in the Clinical Center was beyond the scope of the Marks-Cassell committee, that committee did ask the IC directors to characterize and prioritize their clinical protocols to assess their quality. The criteria used for the assessment included alignment with the NIH and Clinical Center missions, the extent to which the protocol represented cutting-edge science, whether the Clinical Center environment was uniquely appropriate for the study, whether the protocol addressed a national public health emergency, the importance of the protocol for training, whether the protocol was crucial to the institute's research program, whether the protocol was likely to contribute to patient care or patient comfort, and whether the protocol attempted to improve the efficiency or cost effectiveness of patient care. Some of the findings of the assessment—such as that only half of the protocols of NCI's Division of Cancer Therapy, the largest user of the Clinical Center, received excellent or good rankings—led to the identification of programs that were candidates for being phased out.

The present Committee believes that a similar process could be devised for the IRP as a whole to identify programs that represent neither excellent science nor science that is appropriately distinctive for the IRP. They are likely to constitute only a small fraction of the IRP's programs. The identified programs should be considered for phasing out, and the funding associated with them considered for diversion to other high-priority uses, such as trans-NIH projects selected under the proposed NIH strategic planning effort. Opportunities for intramural-extramural collaboration, particularly for clinical research (see Chapter 4) and for research that is capital intensive and requires substantial investments in costly or specialized equipment should also be explored. Such collaborations would improve the IRP's ability to make distinctive contributions to research and NIH should find mechanisms for facilitating and managing them.

The Committee supports the principle that the science conducted by the IRP should be subject to standards of quality similar to those of the extramural program. As noted earlier, the peer review process used to evaluate most extramural research proposals commands widespread respect for its rigorous standards for maintaining research quality. At least some ICs are using comparable peer review for their IRPs. But the peer review process also has a tendency to enforce conservatism by discriminating against research whose outcome is highly uncertain. To evaluate research at the "cutting edge" fairly requires a culture, mindset, and process that views informative failures as the necessary price of strategic innovation. Investigators who conduct projects based on promising but unproven ideas that fail for reasons that could not be foreseen must receive credit for their work. Indeed, the special status of the IRP obligates it to take risks that might not be taken in the extramural program. Such considerations may require novel mechanisms for review, whose adoption could facilitate efforts to distinguish the IRP's role from what can be performed under the current extramural program. It should be reiterated that the Director's Special Projects Program proposed above should be open to ideas from IRP scientists.

The Committee agrees that another important aspect of the IRP is that it is capable of moving quickly and flexibly to meet urgent new needs. There is a lag of about a year while scientists outside NIH apply for and obtain funds to address new topics, but scientists in the IRP can shift focus very quickly simply by electing to do something different. In the middle 1980s, the IRP mounted a major AIDS research program a year before it was possible to award external grants. The importance of that history has again been well illustrated recently as NIAID redirected the efforts of many of its researchers to respond quickly to the threat of bioterrorism and the need for new vaccines and countermeasures; they are also a logical leader in addressing the latest viral epidemic, SARS. NIH's Vaccine Research Center is another example of the IRP filling an important scientific need, for example, by designing a good manufacturing process pilot plant to develop and manufacture large amounts of HIV vaccine candidates for Phase I through Phase III trials. Another example is the high throughput screening program provided by NCI for cancer drug development studies, which is used extensively by academic and industrial laboratories.

Finally, the Committee heard repeatedly that there are historic and cultural factors that have stymied intramural-extramural research collaboration in general. Although there are some notable exceptions, these appear to be more through default than by design. NIH would benefit by promoting the exchange of personnel, space, and resources between the intramural and extramural communities, as appropriate, and as dictated by scientific or health needs.

> Recommendation 8: *Promote Innovation and Risk-Taking in Intramural Research*
> The intramural research program should consist of research and training programs that complement and are distinguished from those in the extramural community and the private sector. The intramural program's special status obligates it to take risks and be innovative. Regular in-depth review of each component of the intramural program should occur to ensure continuing excellence. Allocation of resources to the intramural program should be closely tied to accomplishments and opportunities. Inter-institute and intramural-extramural collaborations should be supported and enhanced.

SUMMARY

Although the Committee is not recommending major changes in the number or structure of NIH's institutes and centers, it concludes that the organization needs to be and can be transformed in other ways to meet its and the nation's scientific and health goals. Most important, the Committee concludes that it is time to begin to redirect, over the next 4-5 years, a small but significant fraction of the NIH budget to a series of strategic trans-NIH initiatives that will be carried out by both the intramural and extramural programs under the auspices of the individual institutes and centers working in partnership. Redirected funds will in many cases profoundly influence the core missions of the ICs. This will require the formalization of a careful, open, and consensus-driven planning process under the direction of the NIH director that should be used to select strategic initiatives, assign responsibilities for them, and elicit commitments of funds from participating units. The Committee commends the current NIH director for undertaking what has been referred to as the Roadmap effort. Congress should formalize the process by charging the director to lead a regular trans-NIH planning process to identify major crosscutting issues and opportunities and to generate a small number of high-priority research initiatives. The process should be periodic—perhaps once every 2 years—and should involve substantial input from the scientific community and the public.

The Committee finds that funding for the operations offices of the NIH director has not kept pace as NIH has expanded and has not grown in proportion to NIH's research budget. OD Operations funding is inadequate for the effective management of the organization and should be increased. The Office of the Director does not have the resources to respond to unexpected needs of NIH as a whole without appealing for support from the ICs. Programmatic offices in OD that were created with specific functions should be assessed for successes and failures and whether these entities should be perpetuated indefinitely. The public process for evaluating proposals to create organizational units described in Chapter 4 should also be applied to programmatic offices in the OD.

Finally, to enhance the quality and innovative nature of NIH's portfolio, the Committee proposes a variety of adjustments in intramural research and the creation of a new program in OD to promote high-risk, high-payoff research.

6

Accountability, Administration, and Leadership

Public accountability and leadership are key aspects of the National Institutes of Health's (NIH's) stewardship of the biomedical enterprise because of the imperatives to maintain public trust, reassure Congress that the public's interest is being served, and ensure that NIH's tactical and strategic objectives for its research and training programs are thoughtfully selected, effectively pursued, and responsive to NIH's research mission, national health concerns, and the need to prepare the next generation of scientists.

Accountability is a critical and challenging aspect of leadership. It is especially challenging for an organization like NIH, which serves a broad array of constituencies and is devoted to research and training, in which outputs can be difficult to measure, market discipline is largely absent, and there is incomplete agreement on what metrics are the most appropriate. On the one hand, too mechanistic a system of accountability may fail to capture the nuances of scientific progress and indeed may stifle it or lead to an illusion of precision. On the other hand, too loose a system of accountability may lead not only to a potential loss of public confidence and trust but also to uncertainty about whether NIH's efforts are achieving, even in an approximate way, its objectives.

This chapter focuses on means by which NIH can enhance its public accountability and ensure the continuing vitality of its leadership, both of which are influenced by and have a capacity to alter the agency's organizational effectiveness. Specifically, the Committee focused on the need for improved NIH-wide data gathering and coordination, increased attentiveness to hiring and review of senior leaders, and better use of the advisory committee system. Important additional aspects of NIH's ability to meet its scientific and public health mission are the availability of sufficient resources in its management-support network to accomplish its goals, and the ability to direct administrative functions in the best interest of its research and training mission.

ANNUAL MECHANISMS FOR PUBLIC ACCOUNTABILITY

Each year, NIH must complete two processes for accounting to Congress and the President on its progress in meeting its goals, conforming to its mission, and justifying its request for appropriations for the next fiscal year. Those processes, developing the budget and responding to the Government Performance and Results Act (GPRA) of 1993, are not sufficient to meet all accountability needs but they do provide useful starting points.

The Budget Process: Congressional Justification

Every fall, each institute or center (IC) with an appropriation must prepare a congressional justification budget (the CJ) that details accomplishments of the preceding year, current initiatives, and plans.[1] The process of preparing the CJ is labor-intensive; programs in each IC are surveyed for data and material considered crucial for justifying programs and budgets. Each IC's information is submitted to the Office of the Director (OD), where it is reviewed and then compiled with all the other IC's CJs and submitted to the Office of Management and Budget (OMB). The exception to this process is the National Cancer Institute (NCI), which under the National Cancer Act of 1971 develops a "bypass budget" that goes directly to the President and OMB.

The budget process is, perhaps, the most powerful accountability mechanism used by NIH, forcing the agency and its various units to justify their places in the programs of the President. It is both a planning and an accountability process. As in other federal agencies, the deadlines of the budget process drive the planning and priority-setting process. In addition, the capacity to influence the congressional appropriation process is one of the major ways in which NIH leadership can coordinate activities across NIH. Thus, development of the annual CJ provides the perfect opportunity for NIH to respond to the Committee's call for more investment in trans-NIH initiatives, as described in Chapter 5. If all ICs were required to account for trans-NIH activities in their CJs, the NIH director, the Secretary of Health and Human Services, and Congress would have a better sense of progress in this category of work.

---

[1]The formal title is "Justification of Estimates for Appropriations Committees." The CJ has a section for each IC, consisting of a set of tables and budget narrative (see Department of Health and Human Services, 2002).

The New Approach to the Government Performance and Results Act

Under GPRA, every major federal agency must ask itself some basic questions every year: What is its mission? What are its goals and how will it achieve them? How can it measure performance? How will it use performance results to make improvements?

GPRA forces a shift in the focus of federal agencies away from such traditional concerns as staffing and activity levels toward a single overriding issue: results. GPRA requires agencies to set goals, measure performance, and report on accomplishments annually. Every NIH IC goes through an annual process in which program managers are asked to review their portfolios for scientific accomplishments that provide evidence of meeting goals and missions.

Until 2003, NIH tracked the success of its programs through a comprehensive overview of its progress by reviewing and compiling scientific advances and external recognition of NIH-supported investigators. Starting in 2003, however, NIH is using more specific and transparent goals to measure research outcomes; the Committee supports this change.

The new framework being used by NIH characterizes goals on the basis of the likelihood that they will be attained and the time targeted for completion. For FY 2004, there are 27 goals arranged according to their likelihood of success and years to completion; the longest time line is set at 10 years (Table 6.1). According to NIH, the goals must be credible to researchers, the public, and other NIH stakeholders and should be as specific as possible to address definable problems. Goals that lend themselves to annual reporting and reports of incremental progress are encouraged. NIH goals must also coordinate with the overall Department of Health and Human Services (DHHS) plan, as well as those of the Centers for Disease Control and Prevention (CDC), the Agency for Healthcare Research and Quality (AHRQ), the Food and Drug Administration, the DHHS "Healthy People 2010" initiative, and the President's Management Agenda.

COUNCIL OF PUBLIC REPRESENTATIVES

NIH created the Council of Public Representatives (COPR) and Public Liaison Offices in response to an Institute of Medicine (IOM) report (IOM, 1998), which recommended that such bodies be created to formalize and systematize communication with the public at the highest levels of NIH. The scope and activities of COPR are evolving, but its charge is broad. COPR is a federal advisory committee of 21 members of the public from across the country who are chosen through an open nomination and application process. Its role is to advise the NIH director on public input and participation in NIH's activities, research priority setting, and outreach programs and efforts. Thus, COPR provides a formal mechanism for public input at the level of the NIH director, but there are multiple additional opportunities for public input across NIH. In addition, each institute has public

TABLE 6.1 NIH GPRA Research Outcomes

RISK	1-3 years	4-6 years	7-10 years
High	1a Conduct medications development with use of animal models, and begin to conduct Phase I and II trials of two potential treatments for alcoholism: cannabinoid antagonist Rimonabant and corticotropin-releasing hormone antagonist Antalarmin. 1b By 2006, develop one or more prototypes for a low-power, highly directional hearing aid microphone to help hearing-impaired persons better understand speech in a noisy background.	2a By 2007, demonstrate the feasibility of islet transplantation in combination with immune tolerance induction for the treatment of type 1 diabetes in human clinical studies. 2b By 2009, evaluate the efficacy of two novel approaches to prevent weight gain and/or treat obesity in clinical trials in humans. 2c Develop methods that can classify at least 75% of proteins from sequenced genomes according to evolutionary origin and biological structure. 2d By 2007, develop an HIV/AIDS vaccine.	3a Identify at least one clinical intervention that will delay the progression, delay the onset, or prevent Alzheimer's disease. 3b By 2010, develop one universal antibiotic effective against multiple classes of biological pathogens. 3c Determine the efficacy of using salivary diagnostics to monitor health and diagnose at least one systemic disease by 2013.

continues

TABLE 6.1 Continued

RISK	1-3 years	4-6 years	7-10 years
	4a By 2005, develop two new animal models to use in research on at least one agent of bioterror.

4b By 2005, develop improved animal models that best recapitulate Parkinson's Disease (PD) based on emerging scientific findings of genetic or environmental influences, or interactions of genes and the environment on the development of PD.

4c By FY 2007, identify 20 small molecules that are active in models of nervous system function or disease and show promise as drugs, diagnostic agents, or research tools. | 5a By 2007, evaluate the efficacy of three new treatments for HIV infection in phase II/III human clinical trials in an effort to identify drugs that are more effective, less toxic, and/or simpler to use than the current recommended HIV treatment regimen.

5b Establish the efficacy of statins in preventing progression of atherosclerosis in children with Systemic Lupus Erythematosis (SLE or lupus).

5c Expand the range of available methods to be used to create, analyze, and utilize chemical libraries, which can be used to discover new medicines. Specifically, use these chemical libraries to discover 10 new and unique chemical structures that could serve as the starting point for new drugs. | 6a Identify the genes that control the risk for the development of age-related macular degeneration and glaucoma in humans.

6b By 2011, assess the efficacy of at least three new treatment strategies for reducing cardiovascular morbidity/mortality in patients with type 2 diabetes and/or chronic kidney disease.

6c By 2012, develop a knowledge base on Chemical Effects in Biological Systems using a "systems toxicology" or toxicogenomics approach. |

continues

TABLE 6.1 Continued

RISK	1-3 years	4-6 years	7-10 years
	7a By 2005, evaluate 10 commonly used botanicals for inhibition/induction of enzymes that metabolize drugs as a method of identifying potential botanical/drug interactions. 7b By 2006, integrate nanotechnology-based components into a system capable of detecting specific biomarker(s) (molecular signatures) to establish proof of concept for a new approach to the early detection of cancer, and, ultimately, cancer preemption. 7c By 2005, create the next generation map of the human genome, a so called "haplotype map" (HapMap), by identifying the patterns of genetic variation across all human chromosomes.	8a By 2007, determine the sequence of an additional 45 human pathogens and three invertebrate vectors of infectious diseases. 8b Identify and characterize two molecular interactions of potential clinical significance between bone-forming cells and components of bone. Such interactions are defined as those having significant impact on the accrual of bone mass or the actual mechanical performance of bone (i.e., fracture resistance in laboratory animals). 8c Build a publicly accessible Collection of Reference Sequences to serve as the basis for medical, functional, and diversity studies. A comprehensive Reference Sequence Collection will serve as a foundation for genomic research by providing a centralized, integrated, non-redundant set of sequences, including genomic DNA, transcript (RNA), and proteome (protein product) sequences, integrated with other vital information for all major research organisms.	9a By 2009, assess the impact of two major Institutional Development Award (IDeA) programs on the development of competitive investigators and their capacities to compete for NIH research funding. 9b By 2010, demonstrate through research a capacity to reduce the total years lost to disability (YLDs) in the U.S. by 10% by: 1) developing treatment algorithms to improve the management of treatment-resistant and recurrent depression and 2) elucidating the mechanisms by which depression influences at least two comorbid physical illnesses (e.g., heart disease, cancer, Parkinson's disease, or diabetes). Major depression is now the leading cause of YLDs in the nation. 9c By FY 2010, identify culturally appropriate, effective stroke prevention programs for nationwide implementation in minority communities.
Low			

Source: National Institutes of Health, 2003.

relations activities with a major focus on communicating with and receiving input from diverse stakeholders.

COPR provides a relatively new opportunity for receiving public input and increasing accountability to a broad constituency. These and other institutional changes within NIH were designed to increase public accountability, although there has been no formal evaluation of the impact of these changes on indicators of public accountability. Furthermore, no criteria have been proposed to assess and monitor public accountability or the effectiveness of mechanisms to improve or assure it at different levels.

CHALLENGES TO ACHIEVING PUBLIC ACCOUNTABILITY

The committee heard anecdotal evidence that priority setting-criteria often are not transparent to the interested public (for example, voluntary health organizations) and that efforts to follow indicators of success have been limited by lack of well-developed data systems suitable for tracking expenditures and research, training, and other NIH-sponsored activities in relation to institutional goals or priorities.

Because the American public is diverse, it is difficult to know what degree of public accountability is achievable at various levels, and how broadly public accountability should be implemented. Likewise, the public is likely to have divided views on what constitutes or fulfills public accountability. Indeed, in practice much of the monitoring of accountability may fall to advocacy organizations, which may or may not represent the diverse views of the spectrum of individuals suffering from various illnesses. Such organizations also might not advocate health research that cuts across diseases; this may lead to tensions over the accountability mechanisms used by Congress and the administration, including for example the level of appropriations for particular ICs, the formation of new ICs, NIH leadership approval, and program and project mandates included in authorizations and report language.

Given the barriers at both levels of translation (described in Chapter 3 and Sung et al., 2003), another challenge to addressing accountability is the weak link between research results on the one hand and public knowledge and perceptions of their significance, potential impact, and NIH's role on the other. Several institute directors told the Committee that when NIH-supported extramural research results are reported, credit is given primarily to the investigators and their institutions without linking them to NIH's support. Giving credit to individual ICs may also minimize the importance of NIH's combined efforts. Thus, media acknowledgment of NIH's role is often minimal or absent, and this can create misleading impressions of NIH's public accountability. NIH officials told the committee that although there is no overarching (NIH-wide) communication plan, efforts are under way to develop one that mirrors the agency's "Roadmap," one that will review research plans from the perspectives of various audiences to determine whether NIH is communicating effectively. There is no doubt that communicating the depth and breadth of NIH's activities and missions is a challenging task, but doing so and doing so with credibility is essential to bolstering public confidence in the agency and enhancing its accountability.

DATA GATHERING AND REPORTING

A related problem in achieving accountability is that, given the large research and training portfolio of NIH, it is difficult to track NIH's many scientific contributions and make information about them available in a manner that is understandable to all constituents. One of the most common types of questions asked by Congress and the public is how much research on specific diseases is being funded? Such data provide only an approximation of the level of effort devoted to objectives, but individuals and groups concerned about specific diseases or health problems often use them as a measure of input and effort to assess aspects of the NIH research and training portfolio of most interest to them. Even NIH officials complained to the Committee that such data are difficult to gather and are usually suspect because each IC uses its own method to estimate its investment. Although senior management at NIH has long recognized that the absence of a standard method for "coding" is a serious problem, no concerted effort to develop one has yet produced results.

NIH officials often point out that statistics on spending by disease may not be very useful precisely because there are no simple relationships between measures of the burden of disease and how NIH allocates funding. Health needs are an important factor, but there is rarely a straightforward one-to-one relationship between health needs and research funding allocations, let alone estimated incidence, prevalence, or burden of disease. Furthermore, the scientific opportunities for progress vary greatly among diseases in sophistication of the current knowledge base, promising lines of inquiry, and availability of sufficient researchers and facilities. Therefore, the amount of research support that can be linked directly to a specific disease not only is difficult to establish but is not by itself an adequate measure of how much or how well NIH is progressing against the disease. Nor does it reflect the potential relevance of basic research to multiple specific diseases (IOM, 1998) in that it is sometimes difficult to know which research is most relevant to the health problem involved.

Despite those challenges, the Committee concludes that the current lack of an information management method and infrastructure to collect, analyze, and report investment data in a timely fashion must be addressed. It is particularly important for NIH leadership to improve the quality and analysis of its data on the allocation of NIH funds by disease for planning and priority-setting purposes. The problem requires the development of an NIH-wide agreement on what to track and publish and a single method for coding data that uses consistent definitions and deals with the uncertainties inherent in counting research that is only related but not directly applicable to a specific topic. Once developed, the statistics should be kept current and their accuracy ensured through quality control. NIH information management must also be improved to meet goals in tracking scientists trained and supported with NIH funds.

NIH is currently instituting substantial upgrades in its business, grant tracking, and clinical research-protocol IT systems, but these upgrades will not address the problem under discussion here. The committee recognizes that developing an additional informatics system to gather data on the nature of NIH's diverse research and training programs consistently and uniformly is likely to be expensive and time-consuming and will require substantial resources and personnel. However, the development of such a system would provide invaluable information to all parties interested in NIH's programs—Congress, other Executive Branch agencies, the public, the research community, and the leadership of NIH itself. Indeed, the effective management of NIH's research and training programs require such a capacity, which therefore would constitute a worthwhile investment. It also would provide the most reliable information for consideration of proposals to add, merge, or eliminate institutes, centers, and offices. Congress, which is likely to be one of the main beneficiaries of an improved information system, should consider the need for additional resources for this purpose in the budget process.

Recommendation 9: *Standardize Data and Information Management Systems*
For purposes of meeting its responsibilities for effective management, accountability, and transparency, NIH must enhance its capacity for the timely collection, thoughtful analysis, and accurate reporting of the nature and status of its research and training programs and public health advances. Data should be collected consistently across institutes and centers and submitted to a centralized information management system.

BUILDING ACCOUNTABILITY THROUGH LEADERSHIP

The vision of the NIH leadership regarding accountability and the procedures and structures that the leadership adopts to enhance it are perhaps the most important ingredients in the complex mix of policies and strategies that enable NIH to meet its responsibilities to all its constituents. Leadership and vision may influence the extent to which accountability is reinforced and implemented at diverse levels of the NIH system, from top management through staff and to individual intramural and extramural investigators.

Although there have been performance plans for IC directors and senior scientists since Director Harold Varmus established them in the 1990s, the current administration has required a formal performance assessment for all supervisory personnel throughout the government. All supervisory personnel at NIH therefore are required to develop a "performance contract" listing the items each person is accountable for, which is the basis of an annual assessment. The NIH director must negotiate his or her performance contract with the Secretary of Health and Human

Services. Likewise the NIH director negotiates a contract with each of the more than 40 people who are his direct reports.

The earlier system for performance plans was general in its approach, but the new contracts are more specific, for example, "increase the prevention and public awareness of diabetes." Relevant items cascade down from the top; for example, the diabetes goal is in the President's contract with the Secretary, who then delegates it to the NIH director, who assigns it to the appropriate senior staff. Thus, the performance contracts are a mechanism for senior management to convey what is important to their subordinates. Outreach and communication factors are major items in the contracts of IC directors.

IC directors are also involved in two other types of review:

- Every 5 years, IC directors are reviewed for their overall performance, including scientific leadership, management of their institute or center, and outreach and communications.
- Every 4 years, IC directors who conduct their own research are evaluated scientifically, as are all intramural scientists. That means that the Board of Scientific Counselors of the institute in which the research is performed oversees the review. Most directors conducting their own research do so in another institute to avoid conflict of interest.

Most senior government officials are in the top ranks of the government service system or in the Senior Executive Service (SES) and are covered by a variety of civil service provisions under Title 5 of the personnel law that protect them from dismissal and loss of rights without considerable effort on the government's part. But salaries for SES personnel are capped. To be able to offer higher salaries and attract the nation's most distinguished scientists, NIH obtained permission 10 years ago to place its senior positions under Title 42 of the law. Title 42 allows NIH to offer higher salaries, although people hired under this authority lose many of the civil service protections provided under Title 5 and must accept 5-year terms as opposed to permanent employment. Most directors chose to move into the Title 42 program, so they are, in fact, already subject to 5-year renewable terms. Under this system the Secretary of Health and Human Services retains approval authority for appointments. Thus, the NIH director can only recommend, but not appoint, senior leadership in the agency. The committee concludes that this lack of authority hinders the ability of the NIH director to form a cohesive senior leadership team to achieve NIH goals.

The committee also concludes that in the current NIH environment, reviews of leadership—a form of public accountability—are too informal and ad hoc to be effective. The processes and criteria for review are not obvious or well defined. One of the more obvious criteria for review, in addition to scientific excellence and leadership skills, should be an individual's performance in imagining and engaging in creative collaborations with colleagues in other institutes and centers, as such collaborations will be an increasingly important aspect of moving some of the most needed new NIH initiatives forward. And the informal review process has changed and depends on the particular policies and practices of the sitting NIH director and the personnel system in which a given IC director resides.

The committee also believes that a healthy degree of turnover in leadership is critical for sustaining the vitality of a research organization. It also provides the opportunity for leading scientists across the nation to leave their positions for a set period and to come to NIH as a form of public service and, in part, to provide effective scientific leadership to critical elements of the nation's biomedical enterprise.

> Recommendation 10: *Set Terms and Conditions for IC Director Appointments and Improve IC Director Review Process*
>
> a. All IC directors should be appointed for 5-year terms. The possibility of a second and final term of 5 years should be based on the recommendation of the director of NIH, which should include consideration of the findings of an external review of job performance. The authority to hire and fire IC directors should be transferred from the Secretary of Health and Human Services to the NIH director.
>
> b. The director of NIH should establish a process of annual review for the performance of every IC director in terms of his or her effectiveness in fulfilling scientific and administrative responsibilities. The results of such reviews should be communicated, as appropriate, to the Advisory Committee to the director and/or the Council of Public Representatives.

By communicating, as appropriate, the results of reviews to the NIH director's advisory groups, the IC directors can demonstrate an additional level of accountability. While some aspects of a review should be held as confidential, those elements that relate directly to the mission and objectives of NIH should be made available to the director's advisors.

The committee concluded that review and revitalization of the OD is an essential prerequisite for accountability and leadership. The committee noted that the National Science Foundation Act of 1950 (42 U.S.C. 1861 et seq.), as amended, creates a term of 6 years for the NSF director and concluded that this has been a good model for creating a system of accountability and periodic review that has the possibility of transcending changes in administrations.

> Recommendation 11: *Set Terms and Conditions for the NIH Director Appointment*
> The NIH director, appointed by the President, should serve for a term of 6 years unless removed sooner by the President. The possibility of a second and final

term of 6 years should be based on a positive external review of performance and the recommendation of the secretary of Health and Human Services.

Finally, the Committee believes that the special status granted NCI by the National Cancer Act should be re-examined. The National Cancer Act of 1971, in addition to making the NCI director a Presidential appointee, created the President's Cancer Panel, composed of two scientists and one management specialist who provide progress reports to the President on the status of NCI's research. The act also replaced the National Cancer Advisory Council with an 18-member National Cancer Advisory Board composed of scientists and laypersons offering guidance and advice to NCI on all major initiatives. In addition, the act allows the NCI director to submit the institute's budget directly to the President, bypassing the NIH director in the process.

Because the President appoints the NCI director and the NCI budget bypasses the NIH director, it is possible that an unnecessary rift is created between the goals, mission, and leadership of NIH and those of NCI. NCI is by far and has been for some time the largest NIH institute (approximately 17% of the total NIH budget). It is not in the interests either of NIH's overall research and training programs, or of NCI, for the NIH director to have such limited authority. In addition, as the biological and cellular basis of cancer becomes more widely understood, the basic science underlying cancer research has direct implications for the etiology and progression of numerous other diseases, for example the autoimmune, infectious, and even cardiovascular diseases. Thus, for scientific and administrative reasons, NCI's special status should be reconsidered.

Recommendation 12: *Reconsider the Status of the National Cancer Institute*
Congress should reassess the provisions of the National Cancer Act of 1971, particularly as they affect the authority of the NIH director to hire senior management and plan and coordinate the NIH budget and its programs in their entirety.

It should be noted that the requirement that NCI prepare a bypass budget every year has some positive aspects in that the institute must undertake an annual strategic planning process. This useful exercise should not be dropped if NCI changes its administrative status as recommended above. Rather, all ICs should be required to develop an annual strategic plan, if they are not already doing so.

THE ADVISORY COMMITTEES

Like other federal science agencies, NIH makes extensive use of advisory committees of nonfederal scientists, health advocacy representatives, and others to ensure the best possible input of expertise and additional perspectives on the evaluation of programs and the development of policies and priorities. NIH had over 140 chartered advisory committees as of May 2002, more than any other federal agency.[2] The Public Health Service Act (PHSA) authorizes appropriate scientific and technical peer review of biomedical and behavioral research grant and cooperative agreement applications, research and development contracts, and research conducted at NIH through its advisory committees.

As described in greater detail in Chapter 2, NIH uses several types of advisory committees. Those groups can be located in the Center for Scientific Review (CSR) (the study sections) or the councils and boards created and used by individual institutes that choose not to use CSR for review of particular initiatives. National Advisory Councils and Boards perform the second level of peer review for research grant applications and offer advice and recommendations on policy and program development, program implementation, evaluation, and other matters of importance for the mission and goals of the IC; and they provide oversight of research conducted by IC intramural programs. The dual review system, which separates the scientific assessment of proposed projects from policy decisions about scientific areas to be supported and the resources to be allocated, permits a more objective evaluation than would result from a single level of review. NIH can make awards only if they have been approved by a national advisory council and the Secretary, and this helps to insulate NIH from pressure by a member of Congress or the administration to fund a particular project. The national advisory councils are also charged with providing advice on policies and programs, although several studies have found that members of the national advisory councils do not always feel they play a strong role in policymaking.[3] The dual system of review provides the responsible NIH officials with advice about both scientific and societal values and needs (NIH, 1992b).[4]

In the appointment process, the President generally follows the recommendations of the Secretary, and the Secretary generally follows the advice of the NIH and IC directors in filling positions, although they add their own candidates from time to time. During the 1972-1974 period, when the Nixon Administration was trying to exert greater control over the NIH budget, there was conflict with the scientific community over the perceived politicization of the advisory committee appointment process; this issue re-emerges from time to time and is of current concern to the scientific and health advocacy communities (e.g., Bass et al., 2003). Moreover as a general matter, the success of any scientific enterprise is dependent on the encourage-

---

[2]They have 4,298 members, 75% of whom are members of initial review groups that evaluate applications for research funding. See overview and list of committees by appointing officials at http://www1.od.nih.gov/cmo/about/index.html.

[3]One study was conducted by the Institute of Medicine's Committee for a Study of the Organizational Structure of the National Institutes of Health in 1984. The other was conducted in the mid-1990s by a committee appointed by the NIH director. Neither report was made public. Copies are in the possession of the authors.

[4]Contracts are subjected to a similar peer review process, except that the second level of review is by senior IC staff.

ment of a wide variety of independent views. The Committee believes that it is essential that members be appointed to these advisory groups because of their ability to provide scientific or public health expertise to the review and approval of awards and policies. They should not be selected to advance political or ideological positions.

Several related issues emerged during the committee's deliberations with respect to NIH's advisory council system. First, there are important differences in the use and roles of the councils among ICs. Some councils are actively involved in setting institute goals and planning. In other cases, council actions are pro forma, with little advice or involvement sought from council by institute personnel. In still other cases, council members might also be grantees of the institute, and thus might feel constrained in expressing strong views or views that differ from than those held by institute or program staff. Those issues highlight a missed opportunity for NIH. Advisory councils should routinely and consistently be consulted in the priority setting and planning processes of an institute. They should have active involvement in decisions regarding issuance of program announcements and requests for applications, which often reflect an institute's priorities and responses to emerging opportunities or demands. They should be working to ensure that the IC is held accountable in reaching its goals and communicating with the public. They should understand and be supportive of relevant trans-NIH initiatives. Finally, a criterion for review of every institute director should be how he or she interacts with and uses the expertise of his or her advisory council.

Under Section 406 of the PHSA, national advisory councils have up to 18 members appointed by the Secretary and nonvoting ex officio members from NIH and other federal agencies. Two-thirds of the appointed members are to be "from among the leading representatives of the health and scientific disciplines (including not less than two individuals who are leaders in the fields of public health and/or social sciences) relevant to the activities of the national research institute" and one-third "from the general public and shall include leaders in the fields of public policy, law, health policy, economics, and management." The Committee believes that the advisory council system should guarantee that ICs receive independent and qualified advice. Their members therefore must be reasonably free of conflicts of interest. In addition, if NIH is to achieve the goal of increased trans-NIH collaborations, it will be important to have cross-fertilization of institutes through advisory council membership. For example, it would be useful to have a cancer researcher (who receives funding from NCI or the American Cancer Society) serve on the council of the National Institute of Environmental Health Sciences or the National Institute of Child Health and Human Development.

Recommendation 13: *Retain Integrity in Appointments to Advisory Councils and Reform Advisory Council Activity and Membership Criteria*

a. Appointments to advisory councils should be based solely on a person's scientific or clinical expertise or his or her commitment to and involvement in issues of relevance to the mission of the institute or center.

b. The advisory council system should be thoroughly reformed across NIH to ensure that these bodies are consistently and sufficiently independent and are routinely involved in priority-setting and planning discussions. Councils should be effectively engaged in discussions with IC leadership to enhance accountability, facilitate translation of goals and activities to the scientific community and the public, and provide feedback to the IC director. To achieve sufficient independence and avoid conflicts of interest, a substantial proportion of a council's scientific membership should consist of persons whose primary source of research support is derived from a different institute or center or from outside NIH.

RESEARCH MANAGEMENT AND SUPPORT

Although administrative or overhead costs are often suspect in the eyes of those who would like to see more money going directly to research or training, at appropriate levels they are essential to the effectiveness of any organization, including those that sponsor research and training programs. Similarly, the effectiveness of those responsible for the wide array of necessary administrative services depends on their leadership and management capabilities and their ability to keep administrative and overhead costs deployed in a manner that best supports the primary missions of the organization.

In the case of NIH, the resources for administrative and overhead functions flow through the Research Management and Support (RMS) budgets of the various units that make up NIH. These budgets, collectively, support all the administrative costs of operating NIH, including management of extramural activities (planning, receipt, peer review, and awards), some intramural research program costs, program development, priority setting, education and outreach, acquisition and maintenance of new information technology systems, professional development, and facility management. Given the structure and funding mechanisms of NIH, the aggregate RMS budget is composed of 25 budget line items, one from each of the ICs that receive separate budget appropriations from Congress. RMS is functionally distinguished from the NIH OD, which is responsible for strategic leadership and receives a separate appropriation.

The administrative costs of NIH have been scrutinized regularly over the last few decades. In the early 1990s, congressional limitations were imposed that restricted inflationary and program growth of the RMS budget. A 1997 management study by Arthur Anderson (National Institutes of Health, 1997b) led to many management improvements, including

- Centralization and improvement of purchasing programs
- Conversion of the mail service to an outsourced performance-based contract

- Development of generic position descriptions
- Hiring of a Chief Information Officer, and
- Creation of a Central Service Review Committee to review the budgets of central service organizations (NIH, unpublished draft report).

In FY 1996, the NIH appropriation contained language that reduced RMS by 7.5% below the FY 1995 level. Despite growth in the overall NIH budget, the RMS reduction was not made up in FY 1997 nor was any growth provided; in FY 1998, an increase of only 1% was allowed. In contrast, from FY 1995 to FY 1999, the extramural program grew at a rate seven times that of RMS. In the FY 2001 budget, RMS represented 3.3% of the total NIH budget, down from 4.5% in 1995. Since FY 1993, the RMS share of the total NIH budget has decreased every year. From FY 1984 through FY 1999, inflation, based on the Gross Domestic Product, increased 58.3%. During the same period, RMS grew 96.2%, while overall NIH grew 217.6%, more than four times the growth rate for RMS (NIH, unpublished draft).

At the same time, the growth in the NIH budget and the rise in congressionally mandated activities have increased the administrative requirements needed to operate a growing and diverse research organization; for example, GPRA is a labor-intensive and expensive annual exercise required by Congress. Other new programmatic requirements have involved the establishment of centers, registries, and other funding requirements, all of which add costs for which RMS must be further stretched.

To accommodate RMS reductions, many institutes have implemented measures to reduce costs, such as introducing modular grant applications and awards, streamlining reviews, and converting to electronic-based research administration. Those are laudable goals under any circumstances, but adverse consequences of the restricted RMS budget seem to be growing. Many are concerned that the strain on the system harms the peer review system, stretches staff too thin, limits business oversight and scientific review, and hinders the ability to respond to increasingly complex research programs and conduct trans-NIH initiatives. NIH's own assessment of the negative impact of the restricted RMS budget found seven areas being adversely affected: stewardship of public funds; scientific advice and program development; public health education and community outreach; information technology acquisition, maintenance, and training; staffing issues; professional development; and facilities management (NIH, unpublished draft). There may have been good reason in the past to celebrate the containment of costs, but the Committee feels that the effectiveness of NIH is now imperiled by the lack of adequate resources to provide appropriate support both for its primary research mission and for meeting its accountability responsibilities.

Other groups have also suggested that RMS funding be raised to provide adequate means for accomplishing NIH's primary goals and to ensure a capacity for strategic planning and evaluation of its programs. In 1998, an IOM committee recommended that Congress "adjust the level of funding for RMS so that NIH can implement improvements in the priority-setting process, including stronger analytical, planning, and public interface capacities" (IOM, 1998). In 2001, the Federation of American Societies for Experimental Biology also recommended increasing RMS. The growing mismatch between the most essential or mandated administrative requirements and the RMS resources available to pay for them must be addressed.

> **Recommendation 14:** *Increase Funding for Research Management and Support*
> Congress should increase the appropriation for RMS to reflect more accurately the essential administrative costs required to effectively operate a world-class $27 billion/year research organization. Moreover, when additional congressional mandates are imposed on NIH through the appropriations process, they should include funds to cover necessary administrative costs.

SUMMARY

NIH uses resources in various ways to enhance public accountability, leadership, and management efficiencies. However, improvements can be made.

First, NIH must commit to developing an improved system for gathering, managing, and reporting data to facilitate public engagement, strategic planning, management of the research and training portfolios, congressional justifications, and scientific communication.

Second, increased attention to the system of hiring and periodic and systematic review of IC directors will revitalize the leadership, invigorate the overall scientific community, and facilitate change and evolution of NIH's mission and goals. The NIH director should have the authority to appoint IC directors, including the director of NCI, with the goal of building a team that shares a vision and a plan. Congress should revisit the special status of NCI to determine whether it continues to meet the needs of the current NIH organization and structure.

Third, leadership must make better use of the advisory committee system, which should be a consistent source of independent advice.

Fourth, in order to operate a world-class research agency, NIH must be provided sufficient resources to support its management needs.

7

Putting Principles into Practice

This study was requested by Congress because of growing concerns that the National Institutes of Health (NIH) is becoming too fragmented to be coordinated adequately to address fundamental changes in science or respond quickly enough to health emergencies. The Committee stands in a long line of bodies convened to review some aspect of NIH's administrative structure. The effectiveness of NIH's organization and the effects of having an increasing number of institutes and centers (ICs) has been a recurring concern for nearly half a century. Many of the blue-ribbon committees, panels, and commissions that have looked at NIH, beginning with the Long Committee in 1955 (NSF, 1955), have concluded that there were enough ICs and recommended against adding new ones. A 1984 Institute of Medicine (IOM) committee acknowledged that new institutes might be necessary under some circumstances but recommended a presumption against establishing them unless specific criteria were met through an orderly process. Despite the judgment of the past review groups that NIH should not add ICs, the net result of the dynamics of NIH's political support has been a steady incremental expansion in the number of major units over the years.

The same review groups have also generally found that NIH is a successful organization, whatever the number of ICs at the time—an indication that proliferation is not necessarily harmful. The importance of health problems, the rich opportunities for research progress in the biomedical and behavioral sciences, and past successes in advancing research and its applications are certainly major factors in explaining the degree of NIH's budgetary and structural growth. Although the present Committee concluded that in some ways NIH as currently structured presents some difficult management and programmatic challenges, it also concluded that, at the current time, widespread consolidation or restructuring would not necessarily be the best way to resolve those challenges. In fact, NIH has been productive in part because it is a federation of many specialized and quasi-independent units, and its complex decentralized structure, which has made NIH effective in responding to research opportunities and public needs, is an important source of its success.

Despite the strength imparted by decentralization, there are circumstances in which organizational, rather than structural, change or some form of administrative modification is desirable. Significant operational changes could improve the strength, responsiveness, vitality, and accountability of NIH, the world's greatest biomedical research agency.

The congressional request for this study set a goal of determining the optimal organizational structure for NIH in the context of 21st century biomedical research science. But the organizational structure of NIH cannot be addressed satisfactorily without considering its mission, some of its key processes, and the scientific, social, and political environments within which its activities take place. The Committee therefore interpreted its mandate to consider aspects of NIH's organizational structure beyond the number of administrative units.

In its charge, the Committee was asked to determine whether there are general principles by which NIH should be organized. As set out in Chapter 1, the Committee concluded that NIH's principal mission is to serve as a mechanism for efficiently and effectively deploying federal resources across a wide array of institutions and individuals in the nation's scientific community to advance the scientific frontier and ensure research training of special relevance to human health needs. It then provided as "principles" nine basic policies or goals that would allow NIH to achieve its mission. Consideration of these nine policies or goals provided the framework for the Committee's response to the remaining questions contained in its charge:

- Does the current structure reflect these principles, or should NIH be restructured?
- If restructuring is recommended, what should the new structure be?
- How will the proposed new structure improve NIH's ability to conduct biomedical research and training, and accommodate organizational growth in the future?
- How would the proposed new structure overcome current weaknesses, and what new problems might it introduce?

POLICIES AND RECOMMENDATIONS

Each basic policy or goal identified by the Committee was explored in the context of NIH's organizational structure to determine whether structure enhanced or impeded efforts to achieve it:

1. The NIH research and training portfolio should be broad and integrated, ranging from basic to applied and from laboratory to population-based, in support of understanding health and how to improve it for all populations. The portfolio should reflect a balance between work in existing highly productive domains or disciplines and high-risk, groundbreaking, potentially paradigm-shifting work. It should be especially responsive whenever scientific opportunity and public health and health care needs overlap.

2. NIH should support research that cuts across multiple health domains and disease categories. This might require special efforts to integrate research across NIH components.

3. The NIH research and training portfolio should make special efforts to address health problems that typically do not attract substantial private sector support, such as prevention, some therapeutic strategies, and many rare diseases.

The Committee made several recommendations aimed at achieving those goals. Most important, it made a case for expanding the role of the director of NIH to lead a trans-NIH planning process to identify major cross-cutting issues and opportunities and generate a small number of major high-priority research initiatives. In addition to continuing generous funding for investigator-initiated research projects, the Committee finds compelling the case for multiyear planning that would mobilize coordinated funding from many ICs for a strategic, but revolving set of high-priority trans-NIH projects. Planning and implementation of such initiatives should involve substantial input from the scientific community and the public, and Congress should ensure the necessary funding to conduct the process. The Committee also recommends that Congress revisit the special status granted the National Cancer Institute (NCI) to determine whether its unique position hinders coordinated planning and programmatic activities.

The Committee proposes the creation of a Director's Special Projects Program to fund the initiation of high-risk, exceptionally innovative research projects offering high potential payoff. Suggestions are made as to how the program should operate and be funded.

To improve the agility and responsiveness of NIH, the Committee recommends that the Office of the Director (OD) be given a more adequate budget to support its management roles or greater discretionary authority to reprogram funding from the earmarked components of its budget when necessary to meet unanticipated needs. The Committee concluded that the authorities of the NIH director should be increased to facilitate more overall planning and control of the NIH research agenda. Moreover, funding for OD Operations has not kept pace as NIH has expanded and has not grown in proportion to NIH's research budget. As a result, the OD is unable to respond to unexpected needs of NIH as a whole without appealing for support from the ICs. In particular, if the NIH director is given the responsibility and authority to conduct NIH-wide planning for trans-NIH initiatives, as recommended in this report, the director's budget will need to be increased to take the costs of such planning into account.

Finally, to enhance the quality and innovative nature of NIH's portfolio, greater attention must be paid to clinical research, with an effort to coordinate across the ICs in their intramural and extramural programs. Some clinical research efforts should be merged.

Efforts must be made to ensure that the intramural programs are of the highest quality and are open to collaboration internally and with the extramural community.

4. The standards, procedures, and processes by which research and training funds are allocated should be transparent to applicants, Congress, voluntary health organizations, and the general public. Moreover, a wide variety of constituencies should have input into the setting of broad priorities.

The Committee concludes that NIH lacks the information management methods and infrastructure needed to collect, analyze, and report data adequately, appropriately, and in a timely fashion. In particular, it is incumbent on NIH leadership to improve the quality and analysis of its data on the allocation of NIH funds by disease for planning and priority-setting purposes. NIH should enhance its capacity for the timely collection, thoughtful analysis, and accurate reporting of the nature and status of its research and training programs. Data should be collected consistently across ICs and submitted to a centralized information management system.

The Committee concluded that NIH is not making the best use of its advisory council system to improve transparency, include a broader community in planning and priority-setting, and assess the effectiveness of its programs. The Committee recommends that the advisory council system be thoroughly reformed to ensure that these bodies are consistently and sufficiently independent and are routinely involved in priority-setting and planning discussions.

5. Extramural research should remain the primary vehicle for carrying out NIH's mission. Open competitive peer review should be the usual mechanism guiding extramural funding decisions.

In general, the Committee concluded that the existing peer review system serves the extramural community well, although it has the potential to deter high-risk research outside the mainstream of scientific consensus. The Committee therefore recommends additional mechanisms to promote such research, such as a Director's Special Projects Program and other measures to increase the responsiveness of NIH when needs call for a more immediate reaction than that typically resulting from extensive peer review. However, any effort to change administrative procedures, e.g., those associated with grants management, should be carefully assessed before being implemented to ensure that changes in the name of efficiency do not thwart NIH's mission.

6. The intramural research program (IRP) is a unique federal resource that offers an important opportunity to enhance NIH's capability to fulfill its mission. It should seek to fill distinctive roles in the nation's scientific enterprise, with appropriate mechanisms of accountability and quality control.

Given the time and resources available for it to complete its task, the Committee did not attempt to systematically evaluate the quality of the IRP. The Committee is, however, convinced that the significant efforts of recent years to reinvigorate the IRP and respond to various advisory committee recommendations have met with considerable success and that there is a promising trend toward improved overall quality in the IRP. The Committee applauds recent efforts to improve the program overall. Nevertheless, the balkanization of the IRP persists because of its multiple institutional budgetary and programmatic lines, which reinforce the "stovepipes" and continue to make it difficult for NIH senior management to ensure that the IRP supports NIH's overall strategies and plans. The Committee suggests that it would be useful to consider mechanisms to foster interactions among the IRPs of the individual ICs, such as large-scale reassignments of space to bring similar programs from individual ICs together to create synergies. Another potentially productive avenue to explore would be to reduce the balkanization of the IRPs by clustering programs that share common themes, approaches, and tools.

In the Committee's view, the IRP should not be merely an internal extension of the extramural community but rather should perform distinctive research that the extramural community cannot or will not undertake. The Committee recommends that each IC's IRP have research and training components that distinguish it from the extramural community while complementing extramural programs and taking advantage of the unique environment provided at NIH for intramural research. Inter-institute and intramural-extramural collaborations should be supported and enhanced.

7. As a world-class science institution, NIH should have state-of-the-art management and planning strategies and tools. A key need is the capability for retrieving comprehensive and interpretable NIH-wide data related to its various objectives.

The effectiveness of NIH as a research agency depends on a wide array of administrative services, the resources for which flow through the Research Management and Support (RMS) budgets of the various NIH units. The allocation for RMS in recent years has been too low for NIH to operate a world-class $27 billion/year research organization and should be increased. The Committee recommends that

Congress increase RMS to reflect more accurately the essential administrative costs that are required to operate NIH effectively. Moreover, when additional congressional mandates are imposed on NIH through the appropriations process, they should include funds to cover necessary administrative costs.

The Committee recognizes that developing the appropriate systems for data collection and management is likely to be an expensive long-term undertaking that will require substantial resources and personnel. However, such a system would provide invaluable information to all parties interested in NIH's programs—Congress, other Executive Branch agencies, the public, the research community, and NIH leadership itself—and therefore would constitute a worthwhile investment. It also would provide the most reliable information for considering any proposals to add, merge, or eliminate institutes, centers, and offices.

8. There should be appropriate mechanisms to ensure the continuing review, evaluation, and appointment of senior scientific and administrative leaders at all levels of NIH.

The vision and skills of NIH leadership are perhaps the most important ingredients in the complex mix of policies and strategies that enable NIH to meet its responsibilities to all its constituents. Moreover, NIH leadership at all levels is responsible for setting goals according to mission, implementing the goals, and assessing progress toward them. Leadership and vision may influence particularly the extent to which accountability is reinforced and implemented at diverse levels of the NIH system, from top management through staff and to individual intramural and extramural investigators. It is the quality of leadership and decision-making, as opposed to administrative structures, that is central to NIH's vitality. In the long run, recruitment of outstanding leaders is essential to NIH's continuing success. The Committee concluded that more rigorous measures are needed to ensure that NIH leadership is periodically revitalized and reviewed. It developed series of recommendations regarding the review and appointment of IC directors, including terms of appointments and the NIH director's authority to make such appointments, and reassessment of the special status of the NCI director. The Committee suggests establishing 6-year terms for the NIH director.

9. Proposals for the creation, merger, or closure of institutes, centers, and offices should be considered through a process of thoughtful public deliberation that addresses potential costs, benefits, and alternatives.

The Committee concluded that, at the current time, the costs of a wholesale consolidation of NIH are likely to outweigh the benefits. Nevertheless, NIH should have sufficient flexibility to consider additions, reductions, or consolidations of NIH administrative units. The NIH director and the public should be able to suggest additions, subtractions, or mergers of units to Congress at appropriate times. However, there should be a formal process for considering proposals for additions, reconfigurations, or reductions that arise from the scientific community, advocacy groups, or Congress. It is not so much the number of units that predicts the success of NIH, but rather the justification of the existence of a given unit and its proven merit. The Committee concludes that there should be a more formal and systematic approach to making changes in NIH's organizational structure. The Committee recommends that on receiving a congressional request or at the discretion of the NIH director in responding to a public request, the director should initiate a public process to evaluate its scientific needs, opportunities, and consequences, the likelihood of available resources, and the level of public support to create a new institute, center, or office, or to consolidate or dissolve units. The Committee does not suggest criteria for making such decisions, as they are likely to change in light of scientific opportunities, fiscal constraints and opportunities, and health needs. But the establishment of an open system by which such decisions are made provides an opportunity for developing criteria case-by case.

SUMMARY

NIH is increasingly called on to undertake research that involves multiple institutes, multiple disciplines, and complex diseases to be responsive to new challenges, such as public health emergencies and the threat of acts of bioterrism. A key question posed to the Committee was whether NIH's decentralized structure has become too fragmented to respond adequately to those challenges or whether, on the contrary, it is well suited to respond to changes in opportunity and need. Related questions included whether, to help equip NIH for the future, the director's authorities should be increased and in what way or whether managerial mechanisms should be strengthened or new ones adopted in place of or in conjunction with structural reorganization.

The Committee's view of those complexities was governed by the desire to be of some practical assistance to all who wish NIH to continue to be an effective—indeed, outstanding—organization. Thus, the Committee proceeded on the premise that its task included assessing the organizational configuration of NIH and the key processes and authorities that play roles in trans-NIH decision-making. Although the borders between structure, mission, and priorities are themselves not well defined, the Committee tried not to take too expansive a view of its responsibilities. It concluded on the one hand that in many ways NIH is performing exceptionally well, using decentralization as a strength. On the other hand, it made multiple recommendations to enhance NIH's vitality and accountability through change, augmentation of existing structures, modifications of policies and practices, and measures that aim to transcend decentralization.

Whether needs and opportunities will be accommodated in existing NIH units or proliferation or consolidation will occur in the near future is an issue to be addressed by administrations, Congress, the scientific community, and the public.

NIH will continue to be shaped by the dynamics of many constituencies interacting. Interests will converge or conflict, depending on the issue. The degree of convergence and divergence will continue to be influenced by other factors such as annual appropriations. The recommendations made in this report are intended to help NIH to continue to be responsive, accountable, and effective in its leading role in the vast international humanitarian enterprise aimed at a better understanding of the human condition, the prevention and relief of the burdens of disease, and at the promotion of good health throughout the stages of life.

References

Association of American Medical Colleges, American Medical Association, and Wake Forest University School of Medicine. (1999). Clinical Research: A National Call To Action. Washington, D.C.

Augustine, N. Member of Committee on the Organizational Structure of the National Institutes of Health, personal communication to Committee, November, 2002.

Bass, G.D., Blumenthal, P.D., Corfman, P. et al. (2003). More on science and politics (letter). Science 299:1313.

Betz, F. Former NSF program officer, personal communication to Gil Omenn, June, 2003.

Biotechnology Industry Organization (BIO). (2003). Biotechnology Industry Statistics. Found on the BIO Internet home page at http://www.bio.org/er/statistics.asp

Botstein, D. (2000). The role of the private sector in training the next generation of biomedical scientists, proceedings of a conference sponsored by the American Cancer Society, the Burroughs Wellcome Fund, and the Howard Hughes Medical Institute, Chevy Chase, Md. (Feb. 14-16).

Burley, S.K. (2000). An overview of structural genomics. Nat Struct Biol. 2000 Nov;7 Suppl:932-4.

Bush, Vannevar. (1945). Science: The Endless Frontier. Washington, D.C.: United States Government Printing Office.

Center for Scientific Review. (1999). "From the CSR Director's Desk," Peer Review Notes, Center for Scientific Review, National Institutes of Health, Bethesda, Md. (September). At http://www.csr.nih.gov/prnotes/sep99prn.htm.

Center for Scientific Review. (2000a). "From the CSR Director's Desk," Peer Review Notes, Center for Scientific Review, National Institutes of Health, Bethesda, Md. (January). At http://www.csr.nih.gov/prnotes/jan00prn.htm.

Center for Scientific Review. (2000b). Panel on Scientific Boundaries for Review, "Phase Report," Center for Scientific Review, National Institutes of Health, Bethesda, Md. (January). At http://www.csr.nih.gov/archives/summary012000.htm.

Center for Scientific Review. (2000c). "From the CSR Director's Desk," Peer Review Notes, Center for Scientific Review, National Institutes of Health, Bethesda, Md. (May). At http://www.csr.nih.gov/prnotes/may2000prn.htm.

Center for Scientific Review. (2000d). "CSR vs. IC Review: Similarities and Differences," Peer Review Notes, Center for Scientific Review, National Institutes of Health, Bethesda, Md. (September). At http://www.csr.nih.gov/prnotes/sep00bod.htm#similar.

Cohen, J. (1993). Conflicting agendas shape NIH. Science 261:1674-1679.

Congressional Budget Office. (2002). Unauthorized appropriations and expiring authorizations. At http://www.cbo.gov/showdoc.cfm?index=3266&sequence=0&from=7.

Cohen, J. J., Hasselmo, N, and Magrath, C.P. (2003). Letter re: National Center for Research Resources 2004 Strategic Plan, 68 FR 4503-4. At http://www.aau.edu/research/Ltr5.9.03.pdf.

Cook-Deegan, R. (1994). Gene Wars. New York: W.W.Norton & Company.

Cook-Deegan, R. (1996). Does NIH need a DARPA? Issues in Science and Technology, winter 1996.

Cooper R.S. (2001). Social inequality, ethnicity and cardiovascular disease. Int J Epidemiol. Oct; 30 Suppl 1:S48-52.

De Tocqueville, Alexis. (2000). Democracy in America. Chicago, Ill.: University of Chicago Press.

Dennis, C. (1999) Varmus speculates on a possible reorganization of the NIH. Nature. 400(5 August 1999):491.

Department of Health, Education, and Welfare. (1958). The Advancement of Medical Research and Education Through the Department of Health, Education, and Welfare. Final Report of the Secretary's Consultants of Medical Research and Education. Washington, D.C.: Government Printing Office.

Department of Health, Education, and Welfare. (1976). Report of the President's Biomedical Research Panel. DHEW Publication (OS) 76-500 and related volumes. Washington, D.C.: Department of Health, Education, and Welfare.

Department of Health and Human Services. (2001). Workforce restructuring plan. November 9.

Department of Health and Human Services. (2002). Justification of estimates for appropriations committee, fiscal year 2003, National Institutes of Health, Volume I.

Drew, E. (1967). The health syndicate: Washington's noble conspirators. Atlantic Monthly Dec. 1967:75-82.

Graham, A.W., and Schultz, T.K., editors. (1998). Principles of Addiction Medicine, 2nd edition. Chevy Chase, Md.: American Society of Addiction Medicine.

Haley, S. (2001). Kirschstein tells how NIH is adapting to the evolving multidisciplinary research model. Washington Fax, May 7, 2001. At http://www.washingtonfax.com.

Hanash, S., and Celis, J.E. (2002). The Human Proteome Organization: A mission to advance proteome knowledge. Mol Cellular Proteomics 1.6:413-414.

Hanson, G.R., and Li, T.H. (2003). Public health implications of excessive alcohol consumption. Journal of the American Medical Assoc. 289(8):1031-1032.

Hawana, J. (2003). Chronic disease cure center Part One of presidential candidate Lieberman's health care plan. Washington Fax May 23, 2003. At http://www.washingtonfax.com.

Helms, W.D. (2002). Funding and Priorities for Health Services Research. Presentation by the President & CEO of the Academy for Health Services Research and Health Policy to the Institute of Medicine's Clinical Research Roundtable, June 12, 2002. Available at http://www.iom.edu/iom/iomhome.nsf/pages/Clinical+Research+Roundtable+June+12+2002+Agenda?OpenDocument

Hood, L. (2003). Systems biology: integrating technology, biology, and computation. Mech Ageing Dev. 124(1):9-16.

Institute of Medicine. (1984). Responding to Health Needs and Scientific Opportunity: The Organizational Structure of the National Institutes of health. Washington, D.C.: National Academy Press.

Institute of Medicine. (1988). A healthy NIH intramural program: structural change or administrative remedies? Washington, D.C.: National Academy Press.

Institute of Medicine. (1998). Scientific Opportunities and Public Needs: Improving Priority Setting and Public Input at the National Institutes of Health. Washington, D.C.: National Academy Press.

Institute of Medicine. (1999). Toward Environmental Justice: Research, Education, and Health Policy Needs. Washington D.C.: National Academy Press.

Institute of Medicine. (2000). Bridging Disciplines in the Brain, Behavioral, and Clinical Sciences. Washington, D.C.: National Academy Press.

Institute of Medicine. (2002). Unequal Treatment: Confronting Racial and Ethnic Disparities in Health Care. Washington D.C.: National Academy Press.

Institute of Medicine. (2003a). Large-scale Biomedical Science: Exploring Strategies for Future Research. Washington D.C.: The National Academies Press.

Institute of Medicine. (2003b). Discussion by NIH Panel on Chronic Pain, meeting of the Board on Neuroscience and Behavioral Health, June 2-3, 2003.

Jenkins, S.C. (2002a). NIH research strategy may trend toward putting the pieces together, Zerhouni testifies. Washington Fax, June 12, 2002. At http://www.washingtonfax.com.

Jenkins, S.C. (2002b). NIH "roadmap meetings" identify trans-agency issues for proactive attention. Washington Fax, October 16, 2002. At http://www.washingtonfax.com.

Kirschstein, R. (2001). Speech at American Institute for Medical and Biological Engineering annual meeting. National Academy of Sciences Auditorium, Washington, D.C., March 1.

Leshner, A., Member of the Committee on the Organizational Structure of the National Institutes of Health, currently Chief Executive Officer, Amercian Association for the Advancement of Science, formerly director, National Institute on Drug Abuse. Personal Communication.

McGeary, M., and P.M. Smith. (2002). Organizational Structure of the National Institutes of Health: Background Paper prepared for the National Academy of Sciences.

Metheny, B. (2002). Accelerated translation of discoveries into practice is a national priority, Zerhouni tells AAMC. Washington Fax November 13, 2002. http://www.washingtonfax.com/.

Miller, G. (2003). Spying on the brain, one neuron at a time. Science 300:78-79.

Morris, Thomas D. (1984). "The Current Organization Structure of the National Institutes of Health," Appendix B in Institute of Medicine, Responding the Health Needs and Scientific Opportunity: The Organizational Structure of the National Institutes of Health. Washington, D.C.: National Academy Press.

Nathan, D.G., and H.E.Varmus (2000). The National Institutes of Health and clinical research: a progress report. Nat. Med. 2000 Nov. 6(11):1201-4.

National Bioethics Advisory Commission. (1999). Research Involving Human Biological Materials: Ethical Issues and Policy Guidance: Volume I, Report and Recommendations of the National Bioethics Advisory Commission. Available at http://www.georgetown.edu/research/nrcbl/nbac/pubs.html.

National Institutes of Health. (1976). Bureau Status for Institutes and Divisions. Memorandum from Leon M. Schwarz, Associate Director for Administration, November 22, 1976. Bethesda, Md.

National Institutes of Health. (1992a). Report of the Task Force on the Intramural Research Program of the National Institutes of Health, transmitted April 13, 1992, to Dr. Bernadine Healy, Director, National Institutes of Health, from Richard D. Klausner, M.D., Chief, Cell Biology and Metabolism Branch, National Institute of Child Health and Human Development, NIH.

National Institutes of Health. (1992b). Orientation handbook for members of scientific review groups. Division of Research Grants. Bethesda, Md.

National Institutes of Health. (1994). The Intramural Research Program: Report of the External Advisory Committee of the Director's Advisory Committee and Implementation Plan and Progress Report. Office of the Director, Bethesda, Md.

National Institutes of Health. (1997a). Report of the NIH Director's Panel on Clinical Research. Report to the Advisory Committee to the NIH Director. Clinical Research Program, Bethesda, Md. At http://www.nih.gov/news/crp/97report/index.htm.

National Institutes of Health. (1997b). Review of NIH Administrative Structure and Costs, Final Report. Arthur Andersen Government Services.

National Institutes of Health. (1999a). Proceedings of the 79th meeting of the advisory committee to the director, December. At http://www.nih.gov/about/director/dec99min.htm.

National Institutes of Health. (1999b). The biomedical information science and technology initiative. Working Group on Biomedical Computing Advisory Committee to the Director, Bethesda, Md.

National Institutes of Health. (2001). Setting Research Priorities at the National Institutes of Health. Originally prepared by the NIH Working Group on Priority Setting, 1997, revised October 2001. At http://www.nih.gov/about/researchpriorities.htm#overview.

National Institutes of Health. (2002). Federal Obligations for Health R&D, by Source or Performer, Fiscal Years 1985-2000. On-line table at http://grants2.nih.gov/grants/award/research/sourfund.htm.

National Institutes of Health. (2003a). Memorandum from Acting Director, Executive Secretariat to IC directors, April 10, 2003: IC Directors' Meeting Highlights. At http://www.nih.gov/icd/od/foia/icdirminutes/icdir041003.htm.

National Institutes of Health. (2003b). Government Performance and Results Act, FY 2004 Annual Performance Plan. Bethesda, Md.

National Institutes of Health. Unpublished draft report of the NIH Research Management and Support Exploratory Committee, *Illuminating the Black Box*. Bethesda, Md.

National Research Council. (2002). Making the Nation Safer: The Role of Science and Technology in Countering Terrorism. Washington, D.C.: The National Academies Press.

National Science Foundation. (1955). Medical Research Activities of the Department of Health, Education and Welfare. Report of the Special Committee on Medical Research Appointed by the National Science Foundation at the Request of the Secretary of Health, Education and Welfare. Washington, D.C.: National Science Foundation.

National Science Foundation. (2002a). Science and engineering indicators—2002. National Science Board, Arlington, Va.: (NSB-02-1).

National Science Foundation. (2002b). Guide to Programs FY 2003—NSF funding opportunities. At http://www.nsf.gov/pubsys.ods/getpub.cfm?gp.

Ochs, N. (2003). Reps. Tauzin and Greenwood launch examination of NIH management/oversight. Washington Fax. March 17, 2003. At http://www.washingtonfax.com.

Office of Management and Budget, Executive Office of the President. (2002). The President's Management Agenda, Fiscal Year 2002. At http://www.whitehouse.gov/omb/budintegration/pma_index.html.

Omenn, G.S. (2000) Public health genetics: an emerging interdisciplinary field for the post-genomic era. Annual Rev Pub Health. 21:1-13.

Omenn, G.S. (2003). Science and technology policies concerning the life sciences. In Nelson S., Lita S. (eds). AAAS Science & Technology Yearbook (in press).

Pennisi, E. (2003). Human Genome: Reaching Their Goal Early, Sequencing Labs Celebrate. Science 300(5618): 409.

Pharmaceutical Research and Manufacturers of America. (2001). Pharmaceutical Industry Profile 2001. Washington, D.C.: Pharmaceutical Research and Manufacturers of America.

Pradhan, A.D., J.E. Manson, J.E. Rossouw, D.S. Siscovick, C.P. Mouton, N. Rifai, R.B. Wallace, R.D. Jackson, M.B. Pettinger, and P.M. Ridker. (2002). Inflammatory biomarkers, hormone replacement therapy, and incident coronary heart disease: prospective analysis from the women's health initiative observational study. JAMA. 288:980-987.

Rich, M.W. (2002). From clinical trials to clinical practice: bridging the GAP. JAMA, 287(10): 1321-3.

Sclar, E. (2000). You Don't Always Get What You Pay For: The Economics of Privatization. Ithaca, N.Y.: Cornell University Press,

Silverstein, S.C. (2001). Perspectives from genomics and informatics to medical practice. Issues in Science and Technology, NAS, NAE. Fall:37-41.

Stokes, Donald. (1997). Pasteur's Quadrant. Washington, D.C.: The Brookings Institute.

Sung, N.S., W.F. Crowley, M. Genel, P. Salber, L. Sandy, L.M. Sherwood, S.P. Johnson, V. Catanese, H. Tilson, K. Getz, E.L. Larson, D. Scheinberg, E.A. Reece, H. Slavkin, A. Dobs, J. Grebb, R.A. Martinez, A. Korn, and D. Rimoin. (2003). Central Challenges Facing the National Clinical Research Enterprise. J. Amer. Med. Assoc. 289:1278-1287.

U.S. Congress. (1981). National Institute on Arthritis and Musculoskeletal Diseases—Establishment of, Hearing before Senate Committee on Labor and Human Resources, 97th Congress, 2nd Session, on S. 1939, To amend the Public Health Service Act to establish a National Institute on Arthritis and Musculoskeletal Diseases, July 20. Serial 98-079. Washington, D.C.: U.S. Government Printing Office.

U.S. House of Representatives. 1976. Investigation of the National Institutes of Health, report prepared by the staff of the Committee on Interstate and Foreign Commerce and its Subcommittee on Health and the Environment, 94th Congress, 2nd Session. Washington D.C.: U.S. Government Printing Office.

Varmus, H. (2001). Proliferation of the National Institutes of Health. Science 291:1903-1905.

Waterman, Jr., R.H., Peters, T.J., and Phillips, J.R. (1980). Structure is not organization. Business Horizons 23:14.

Wyngaarden, J.B. (1979). The clinical investigator as an endangered species. N. Engl. J. Med. 301(23):1254-9.

Yen, I.H., Ragland, D.R., Greiner, B.A., Fisher, J.M. (1999). Workplace discrimination and alcohol consumption: findings from the San Francisco Municipal Health and Safety Study. Ethn. Dis. Winter 9(1):70-80.

Appendix A

Sources of Information Provided to the Committee

ORGANIZATIONS

Alliance for Aging Research
American Academy of Allergy, Asthma, and Immunology
American Academy of Head and Neck Surgery
American Academy of Ophthalmology
American Academy of Optometry
American Academy of Orthopaedic Surgeons
American Association for Dental Research
American Autoimmune Related Diseases Association, Inc.
American College of Allergy, Asthma, and Immunology
American Dental Association
American Dental Education Association
American Diabetes Association
American Heart Association
American Obesity Association
American Optometric Association
Arthritis Foundation
Association of American Medical Colleges
Association for Research in Vision and Ophthalmology
Association of Schools of Public Health
Association of University Professors of Ophthalmology
College on Problems of Drug Dependence, Inc.
Epilepsy Foundation

Federation of American Societies of Experimental Biology
Friends of the NIDCR
Institute of Ophthalmology and Visual Science, New Jersey Medical School
International Longevity Center
National Alliance for Eye and Vision Research
National Foundation for Ectodermal Dysplasias
National Mental Health Association
Ohio State University Health Sciences Center
Research Society on Alcoholism
Sjogren's Syndrome Foundation
Society for Women's Health Research
The Ohio State University College of Optometry
The Smith Kettlewell Eye Research Institute
Vision Share

INDIVIDUALS

Sarah Caddick, Steven and Michele Kirsch Foundation
Robert Core and James O'Rourke, University of Connecticut Health Center
William Crowley, Academic Health Centers' Clinical Research Forum
Cedric Garland, University of California, San Diego, School of Medicine
Morton Goldberg, The Wilmer Ophthalmological Institute
Frederick Goodwin, former director, NIMH and ADAMHA
Sandra Hanneman, Texas Medical Center
Bernadine Healy, former director, NIH
Stephen Lippard, Massachusetts Institute of Technology, Department of Chemistry
John Porter, former US Representative
Bob Roehr, Council of Public Representatives at NIH
Louis Sullivan, Morehouse School of Medicine
Thomas W. Stone, Retina and Vitreous Associates of Kentucky
Harold Varmus, former director, NIH
Max Harry Weil, USC School of Medicine and Northwestern University Medical School
Robert D. Wells, Texas Medical Center

DEPARTMENT OF HEALTH AND HUMAN SERVICES

- Robert Wood, Chief of Staff
- Laura Lawlor, Deputy Chief of Staff

NIH Officials—Office of the Director, NIH

- Elias Zerhouni, Director, NIH

- Wendy Baldwin, Deputy Director for Extramural Research
- John Burklow, Office of Communications and Public Liaison
- Stephen Ficca, Associate Director for Research Services
- John Gallin, Director, Clinical Research Center
- Michael Gottesman, Deputy Director for Intramural Research
- Robin Kawazoe, Director, Office of Science Policy and Planning
- Raynard Kington, Director, Office of Behavioral and Social Sciences Research
- Ruth Kirschstein, Deputy Director
- Charles Leasure, Deputy Director for Management
- Donald Poppke, Acting Associate Director for Budget
- Belinda Seto, Acting Deputy Director for Extramural Research Director
- Lana Skirboll, Director, Office of Science Policy

NIH Officials—Institute and Center Directors

- Ellie Ehrenfeld, Director, Center for Scientific Review
- Andrew von Eschenbach, National Cancer Institute
- Paul A. Sieving, Director; Jack A. McLaughlin, Deputy Director; and Michael P. Davis, Associate Director for Science Policy and Legislation, National Eye Institute
- Claude Lenfant, National Heart, Lung, and Blood Institute
- Francis Collins, National Human Genome Research Institute
- Raynard Kington, Acting Director, National Institute on Alcohol Abuse and Alcoholism
- Anthony Fauci, National Institute of Allergy and Infectious Disease
- Richard Hodes, National Institute on Aging
- Steve Katz, National Institute of Arthritis and Musculoskeletal and Skin Diseases
- Duane Alexander, National Institute of Child Health and Human Development
- James Battey, National Institute on Deafness and Other Communication Disorders
- Allen Spiegel, National Institute of Diabetes and Digestive and Kidney Diseases
- Glen Hanson, National Institute on Drug Abuse
- Ken Olden, National Institute of Environmental Health Sciences
- Richard Nakamura, Acting Director, National Institute of Mental Health
- Audrey Penn, Acting Director; Eugene Major, Acting Deputy Director; and Constance Atwell, Director, Division of Extramural Research, National Institute of Neurological Disorders and Stroke
- Patricia Grady, National Institute of Nursing Research

OTHER GOVERNMENT OFFICIALS

- Anthony J. Tether, Director, Defense Advanced Research Projects Agency
- Michael Goldblatt, Director, Defense Sciences Office, Defense Advanced Research Projects Agency

APPENDIX B

Acronyms and Abbreviations

AAMC	Association of American Medical Colleges
AAU	Association of American Universities
ACC	Autism Coordinating Committee
ACD	Advisory Committee to the Director
ADAMHA	Alcohol, Drug Abuse, and Mental Health Administration
AHRQ	Agency for Healthcare Research and Quality
AIDS	Acquired immune deficiency syndrome
ARAC	Administrative Restructuring Advisory Committee
CDC	Centers for Disease Control and Prevention
cDNA	Complementary DNA
CGAP	Cancer Genome Anatomy Project
CIT	Center for Information Technology
CJ	Congressional Justification Budget
COPR	Council of Public Representatives
CSR	Center for Scientific Review
DARPA	Defense Advanced Research Projects Agency
DHHS	Department of Health and Human Services
DOD	Department of Defense
EAC	External Advisory Committee of the Director's Advisory Committee

FDA	Food and Drug Administration
FIC	Fogarty International Center for Advanced Study in the Health Sciences
FY	Fiscal Year
GCRC	General Clinical Research Center
GPRA	Government Performance and Results Act
GS	Government Service
HGP	Human Genome Project
HIPAA	Health Insurance Portability and Accountability Act
HUPO	Human Proteome Organization
IC	Institutes and centers
IOM	Institute of Medicine
IRG	Integrated/Initial Review Group
IRP	Intramural Research Program
MGC	Mammalian Gene Collection
NASULGC	National Association of State Universities and Land Grant Colleges
NCI	National Cancer Institute
NCCAM	National Center for Complementary and Alternative Medicine
NCMHD	National Center on Minority Health and Health Disparities
NCRR	National Center for Research Resources
NEI	National Eye Institute
NHLBI	National Heart, Lung, and Blood Institute
NHGRI	National Human Genome Research Institute
NIA	National Institute on Aging
NIAAA	National Institute on Alcohol Abuse and Alcoholism
NIADDK	National Institute of Arthritis, Diabetes, and Digestive and Kidney Diseases
NIAID	National Institute of Allergy and Infectious Diseases
NIAMS	National Institute of Arthritis and Musculoskeletal and Skin Diseases
NIBIB	National Institute of Biomedical Imaging and Bioengineering
NICHD	National Institute of Child Health and Human Development
NIDA	National Institute on Drug Abuse
NIDCD	National Institute on Deafness and Other Communication Disorders
NIDCR	National Institute of Dental and Craniofacial Disorders
NIDDK	National Institute of Diabetes and Digestive and Kidney Diseases
NIEHS	National Institute of Environmental Health Sciences
NIGMS	National Institute of General Medical Sciences
NIH	National Institutes of Health (National Institute of Health 1930-1948)

NIMH	National Institute of Mental Health
NINCDS	National Institute of Neurological and Communicative Disorders and Stroke
NINDB	National Institute of Neurological Diseases and Blindness
NINDS	National Institute of Neurological Disorders and Stroke
NINR	National Institute of Nursing Research
NIOSH	National Institute for Occupational Safety and Health
NLM	National Library of Medicine
NSF	National Science Foundation
OAM	Office of Alternative Medicine
OAR	Office of AIDS Research
OBB	Office of Bioengineering and Bioimaging
OBSSR	Office of Behavioral and Social Sciences Research
OD	Office of the Director
ODP	Office of Disease Prevention
ODS	Office of Dietary Supplements
OMAR	Office of Medical Applications of Research
OMB	Office of Management and Budget
ORD	Office of Rare Diseases
ORMH	Office of Research on Minority Health
ORWH	Office of Research on Women's Health
PA	Program announcement
PhARMA	Pharmaceutical Research and Manufacturers of America
PHS	Public Health Service
PHSA	Public Health Service Act
P.L.	Public Law
R&D	Research and development
R01	Traditional individual investigator research grant
RFA	Request for application
RMS	Research Management and Support
SARS	Severe Acute Respiratory Syndrome
SEP	Special Emphasis Panel
SES	Senior Executive Service
SGER	Small Grants for Exploratory Research
WHI	Womens' Health Initiative

Appendix C

Committee Member Biographies

Harold T. Shapiro, PhD, Princeton University (IOM), is President Emeritus of both the University of Michigan and Princeton University. He is currently Professor of Economics and Public Affairs, Department of Economics and the Woodrow Wilson School of Public and International Affairs, Princeton University. His research interests include bioethics, the social role of higher education, hospital/medical center administration, university administration, econometrics, statistics, and economics. Shapiro's professional activities include memberships in the Conference Board Inc. and The Bretton Woods Committee. A trustee of the Alfred P. Sloan Foundation (where he is chair of the board), the University of Pennsylvania Medical Center, the Universities Research Association, and the Educational Testing Service, he also serves as a director of the Dow Chemical Company. He is a member of the Institute of Medicine and chaired its 1988 study on "A Healthy NIH Intramural Program: Structural Change or Administrative Remedies?" He is also a member of the American Philosophical Society and a fellow of the American Academy of Arts and Sciences. In July 1996, Shapiro was appointed by President Clinton to chair the National Bioethics Advisory Commission, which issued the report "Cloning Human Beings" in June 1997. From 1990 to 1992, he was a member and vice chair of President Bush's Council of Advisors on Science and Technology. He chaired the Institute of Medicine's Committee on Employer-Based Health Benefits whose report, "Employment and Health Benefits: A Connection at Risk," was published in March 1993. He earned a PhD in economics from Princeton University.

Norman R. Augustine, PhD, Lockheed Martin (NAE), retired in 1997 as Chair and CEO of the Lockheed Martin Corporation and previously served as Chair and CEO of the Martin Marietta Corporation. Upon retiring he served on the faculty of the Department of Mechanical and Aerospace Engineering at Princeton University. Earlier in his career he had served as Under Secretary of the Army and prior to that as Assistant Director of Defense Research and Engineering. Augustine has been Chairman of the National Academy of Engineering, President of the Boy Scouts of America and served nine years as Chairman of the American Red Cross. He has also been President of the American Institute of Aeronautics and Astronautics and served as Chairman of the "Scoop" Jackson Foundation for Military Medicine. He has been a Trustee of MIT, Johns Hopkins and Princeton. He has served on the President's Council of Advisors on Science and Technology and is a former Chairman of the Defense Science Board. He is a member of the American Philosophical Society and is a fellow of the American Academy of Arts and Sciences. His corporate board memberships are Black and Decker, Lockheed Martin, Procter and Gamble, and ConocoPhillips. He has been presented the National Medal of Technology and the Department of Defense's highest civilian award, the Distinguished Service Medal, five times. Mr. Augustine holds an MSE in Aeronautical Engineering from Princeton University and has authored and co-authored four books.

J. Michael Bishop, MD (NAS, IOM), is the Chancellor of the University of California, San Francisco. He won the Nobel Prize together with UCSF colleague Harold Varmus for their discovery of the cellular origin of retroviral oncogenes. Their research has had significant influence on contemporary knowledge about tumor development and the systems that govern cell growth. Bishop is a professor in the departments of microbiology and immunology and biochemistry and biophysics at the University of California at San Francisco. In 1996, he chaired a committee that reviewed the intramural program of the National Cancer Institute. He is a member of the National Academy of Sciences and the Institute of Medicine.

James R. Gavin, III, MD, PhD, Morehouse School of Medicine, is President of Morehouse School of Medicine in Atlanta, Georgia. Prior to his presidency, Dr. Gavin was the senior scientific officer at the Howard Hughes Medical Institute (HHMI) and director of the HHMI-National Institutes of Health Research Scholars Program. He earned his PhD in biochemistry from Emory University in Atlanta in 1970 and his MD from Duke University School of Medicine in 1975. Prior to joining the senior staff of HHMI, he was on faculty at the University of Oklahoma Health Sciences Center as a professor and as chief of the Diabetes Section, acting chief of the Section on Endocrinology, Metabolism and Hypertension, and William K. Warren Professor for Diabetes Studies. He previously served as associate professor of Medicine at Washington University School of Medicine in St. Louis. He was a lieutenant commander in the U.S. Public Health Service (USPHS) from 1971-73 and continues to serve as a reserve officer in the USPHS. Dr. Gavin belongs to a number of organizations, including the Institute of Medicine, the American Diabetes Association, the American Society of Clinical Investigation, the American Association of

Physicians, the Alpha Omega Alpha Medical Honor Society, the Association of Black Cardiologists, Omicron Delta Kappa Honorary Society and the Sigma Pi Phi Leadership Fraternity. He is a past president of the American Diabetes Association (ADA) and was voted Clinician of the Year by ADA in Diabetes in 1991. He has served on many advisory boards and on the editorial boards of the American Journal of Physiology and the American Journal of Medical Sciences. He is on the board of trustees for Duke University, Microislets, Inc., the Robert Wood Johnson Foundation, and is chairman of the board of the Equidyne Corporation. He is national program director of the Minority Medical Faculty Development Program of the Robert Wood Johnson Foundation. He has published more than 180 articles and abstracts in such publications as Science, Journal of Applied Physiology, Diabetes, and the American Journal of Physiology. Among the many honors Dr. Gavin has received are the Daniel Hale Williams Award, the E.E. Just Award, the Herbert Nickens Award, the Daniel Savage Memorial Award, the Emory University Medal for Distinguished Achievement, the Banting Medal for Distinguished Service from the American Diabetes Association, the Distinguished Alumni Award from the Duke University School of Medicine, and the Internist of the Year from the National Medical Association.

Alfred G. Gilman, MD, PhD, University of Texas Southwestern Medical Center (NAS, IOM), is Professor and Chairman of the Department of Pharmacology at the University of Texas Southwestern Medical Center. His research focus is in biochemistry and pharmacology. He won the Nobel Prize in Physiology and Medicine with Martin Rodbell for their discovery of G-proteins and the role of these proteins in signal transduction in cells. He received his MD and PhD in pharmacology from Case Western Reserve University.

Martha Hill, RN, PhD, FAAN, Johns Hopkins University School of Nursing (IOM), is Dean and professor at the Johns Hopkins University School of Nursing. She holds joint appointments in the Bloomberg School of Public Health and the School of Medicine. Dr. Hill, the 1997-1998 president of the American Heart Association, is a Fellow in the American Academy of Nursing and a member of the Institute of Medicine. She served as the Co-vice chair of the recently released IOM Report Unequal Treatment: Confronting Ethnic and Racial Disparities in Health Care. Dr. Hill received her Bachelor of Science degree in nursing from Johns Hopkins University, her masters degree from the University of Pennsylvania, and her doctoral degree in behavioral sciences from the Johns Hopkins University School of Public Health. Dr. Hill is internationally known for her work and research in preventing and treating hypertension and its complications among underserved blacks, particularly among young, urban black men. She is an active investigator and consultant on several NIH funded clinical trials. She has published extensively and serves on numerous review panels, editorial boards, and advisory committees including the Board of Directors of Research!America and the Executive Council of the American

Society of Hypertension. Dr. Hill has also consulted on hypertension and other cardiovascular-related issues outside of the US, including Scotland, Israel, Australia, and South Africa.

Debra Lappin, JD, Princeton Partners, Ltd., served on the NIH Director's Council of Public Representatives from 1999 to 2003. While on the COPR, she chaired its working group on Human Research Protections, served on ad hoc advisory committees addressing NIH Oversight of Human Gene Transfer Research and Trans-NIH Pediatric Research, and provided a "public perspective" of clinical research issues in a number of national settings. Ms. Lappin has served as a member of the Advisory Committee for the National Institute of Arthritis, Musculoskeletal and Skin Disease, as a participant in the Institute of Medicine's public forum examining Clinical Research in the Public Interest, as a member of the IOM Committee addressing Changing Health Care Systems and Rheumatic Diseases, and as a member of an advisory committee at the Agency for Healthcare Research and Quality to examine future directions for the Center for Outcomes and Effectiveness Research. From 1996 to 1998, Ms. Lappin was the Chair of the Arthritis Foundation. Under her leadership, the Arthritis Foundation entered in a partnership with the Centers for Disease Control and Prevention to create the National Arthritis Action Plan, and into a collaborative alliance with Robert Wood Johnson Family Interests to create the Alliance for Lupus Research. Today Ms. Lappin remains active as an Emeritus Trustee of the Arthritis Foundation, lectures as an adjunct faculty member in the Department of Medicine at the University of Colorado Health Sciences Center, and as the President of Princeton Partners, Ltd., consults with academic, industry and non-profit clients in areas of science policy and collaborative partnerships.

Alan I. Leshner, PhD, American Association for the Advancement of Science (IOM), is Chief Executive Officer of the American Association for the Advancement of Science (AAAS) and Executive Publisher of Science magazine. From 1994-2001, he was Director of the National Institute on Drug Abuse at NIH, and from 1988-1994 he was Deputy Director and Acting Director of the National Institute of Mental Health. Prior to that, he spent nine years at the National Science Foundation, where he held a variety of senior positions, focusing on basic research in the biological, behavioral, and social sciences, and on science education. He began his career at Bucknell University, where he was Professor of Psychology. His research has focused on the biological bases of behavior, particularly the role of hormones in the control of behavior. Dr. Leshner is a member of the Institute of Medicine and a fellow of AAAS and many other professional societies. He has received numerous awards from both professional and lay groups for his national leadership in science, mental illness and mental health, and substance abuse and addiction.

Gilbert S. Omenn, MD, PhD, University of Michigan (IOM), is Professor of Internal Medicine, Human Genetics, and Public Health at the University of Michigan. From

1997 to 2002 he was also UM Executive Vice President for Medical Affairs and Chief Executive Officer of the University of Michigan Health System. Previously he was professor of medicine and environmental health and Dean of the School of Public Health & Community Medicine at the University of Washington. He served as Associate Director of the White House Office of Science and Technology Policy and then the Office of Management and Budget in the Carter Administration, and chaired the Presidential/Congressional Commission on Risk Assessment and Risk Management from 1994-97. He has been a National Institutes of Health Research Career Development Awardee, a Howard Hughes Medical Institute Investigator, and founding director of the University of Washington Robert Wood Johnson Clinical Scholars Program. His research is focused on proteomics and cancer prevention, as well as health promotion for older adults, science-based risk analysis, and the ethical, legal, and public health policy aspects of genetics. Dr. Omenn holds an MD from Harvard and a PhD in genetics from the University of Washington.

Franklyn G. Prendergast, PhD, Mayo Cancer Center, is Director of the Mayo Clinic Cancer Center in Rochester, Minnesota, and Professor of Biochemistry and Molecular Biology. His research focus is in structural protein biology and bioimaging. He is a recipient of the E.E. Just award of the American Society of Experimental Biology. He is a member of the American Association for the Advancement of Science, the American Society for Biochemistry and Molecular Biology, and Sigma Xi. He earned his PhD in biochemistry from the University of Minnesota and his medical degree from the University of the West Indies.

Stephen J. Ryan, MD, University of Southern California (IOM), is Professor of Ophthalmology and Dean, Keck School of Medicine of USC and Senior Vice President for Medical Care, University of Southern California. His research relates to macular degeneration, ocular trauma, retinal detachment, and other retinal diseases. He previously served as Chairman of the Department of Ophthalmology at USC and as a member of the National Advisory Eye Council for the NEI of the NIH. He is a member of the Institute of Medicine and currently serves as President of the National Alliance for Eye and Vision Research. He earned his MD from Johns Hopkins University.

Samuel C. Silverstein, MD, Columbia University (IOM), is John C. Dalton Professor of Physiology and Cellular Biophysics and Professor of Medicine at the Columbia University College of Physicians and Surgeons. His research focuses on structure and function of polymorphonuclear and mononuclear leukocytes and endothelial cells in innate immunity, in diseases associated with chronic inflammation such as atherosclerosis and Alzheimer's disease; and in host defense against infectious microorganisms including Legionella pneumophila and M. tuberculosis. He has served on the Councils of the American Society for Cell Biology (1988-92), and the National Institute of Allergy and Infectious Diseases (1995-98) and as President of FASEB

(1994-95). He is a Director of the Cancer Research Fund of the Damon Runyon Foundation and of Research!America; and is President of Funding First, the medical and health research policy program of the Mary Lasker Charitable Trust. Dr. Silverstein is a graduate of Dartmouth College with an AB in government, and of Albert Einstein College of Medicine, where he earned his MD. He is a member of The Institute of Medicine and of the American Academy of Arts and Sciences.

Harold C. Slavkin, DDS, (IOM), is Dean of the School of Dentistry at USC. He previously served as director of the National Institute of Dental and Craniofacial Research, NIH. Under his direction, NIDCR spearheaded many advances and explored a broadening range of research topics, including oral cancer, the genetic causes of craniofacial defects, the link between oral and systemic diseases, biomimetics and tissue engineering. Slavkin is one of the world's leading authorities on craniofacial development and genetic birth defects. Slavkin was founding director of the School of Dentistry's Center for Craniofacial Molecular Biology and was the first holder of the school's George and Mary Lou Boone Chair in Craniofacial Molecular Biology. He earned his DDS from USC.

Judith L. Swain, MD, Stanford University (IOM), is Chair, of the Department of Medicine, Stanford University. Her research focus is in molecular cardiology and angiogenesis, and she pioneered the use of transgenic animals to understand the genetic basis of cardiovascular development and disease. She is a member of the Institute of Medicine, and has served as President of the American Society of Clinical Investigation. She has been a member of two NIH Advisory Councils—National Heart Lung and Blood Institute and the National Research Resources Council—and served as Director of the NIH US/Russia Cardiovascular Biology Program. She currently serves as a member of the Defense Science Research Council of the Defense Advanced Research Project Agency (DARPA). She completed her MD at University of California, San Diego.

Lydia Villa-Komaroff, PhD Whitehead Institute, is Vice President for Research and Chief Operating Officer of the Whitehead Institute for Biomedical Research. Her research interests include molecular aspects of cell biology, academic administration, and biotechnology. Deeply committed to the recruitment and retention of minorities in science, Dr. Villa-Komaroff is a founding member and past officer of the Society for the Advancement of Chicanos and Native Americans in Science. She was Vice President for Research at Northwestern University and served as a member of the Advisory Committee for the Biology Directorate of the National Science Foundation and as a member of the NAS Committee on Assessing the System for Protecting Human Research Participants. She is currently on the boards of the American Association for the Advancement of Science and the National Advisory Council of the National Institute for Neurological Diseases and Stroke. She earned her PhD in cell biology from the Massachusetts Institute of Technology.

Robert H. Waterman, Jr., The Waterman Group, is Founder and Chairman of the Waterman Group, Inc., a management research, writing, and venture management firm. Probably best known as coauthor of *In Search of Excellence*, Waterman is also author of *The Renewal Factor, Adhocracy: The Power to Change*, and *What America Does Right*. Between 1964 and 1985 Waterman was with McKinsey & Company, Inc., where he became a senior director working mainly in California, Australia, and Japan. Waterman currently is chairman of the board of the RLS (Restless Leg Syndrome) Foundation, serves on the NINDS Council, and is a member of the President's Council of the Academy of Sciences and the Board of the World Wildlife Fund. In the past Waterman has served on a variety of public company boards (McKesson, AES, Boise Cascade) and a variety of non-profit boards (San Francisco Symphony, US Ski Team, Center for Excellence in Non-Profit Management).

Myrl Weinberg, CAE, National Health Council, is president of the National Health Council, an umbrella organization that has served as the place where "the health community meets" for 82 years. The Council's 117 members are national organizations that are committed to quality health care, and its core constituency of more than 50 of the leading voluntary health agencies represent approximately 100 million people with chronic diseases and/or disabilities. Ms. Weinberg has a long history of board and committee service, including serving as a member of the Institute of Medicine's Health Sciences Policy Board, Roche Genetics Science and Ethics Advisory Committee, NCQA Committee on Performance Measurement, and as chair of the American Medical Association's Ethical FORCE initiative. In addition, Ms. Weinberg serves as vice chair of the Governing Board of the International Alliance of Patients' Organizations. Ms. Weinberg also served on the congressionally-mandated Institute of Medicine Committee created to assess how research priorities are established at the National Institutes of Health. Ms. Weinberg pursued advanced graduate study at Purdue University. She holds an MA in Special Education from George Peabody College and a BA in Psychology from the University of Arkansas.

Kenneth B. Wells, MD, University of California, San Francisco (IOM), is Professor-in-Residence of Psychiatry and Biobehavioral Sciences at the UCLA Neuropsychiatric Institute (NPI), and a psychiatrist and health services and policy researcher. Dr. Wells directs the UCLA-NPI Health Services Research Center, which focuses on improving quality of care for psychiatric and neurologic disorders across the life span. He also directs training of psychiatrists in health services research and is the Principal Investigator and Director of the NIMH-UCLA-NPI Faculty Scholars Program in mental health services research and Associate Director of the UCLA School of Medicine's Clinical Scholars Program, funded by the Robert Wood Johnson Foundation. He is a member of the Institute of Medicine. He holds an MD from the University of California, San Francisco and an MPH from UCLA.

Mary Woolley, MA, Research!America (IOM), is President of Research!America, a nonprofit public education and advocacy organization committed to making medical and health research a much higher national priority. She began her career in the then largest-ever NIH-supported clinical trial, the Multiple Risk Factor Intervention Trial. Following that, she served as CEO of the Medical Research Institute of San Francisco and as President of the Association of Independent Research Institutes. For her work on behalf of medical research, she has been awarded the Distinguished Contribution to Research Administration Award from the Society of Research Administrators, the Columbia University College of Physicians and Surgeons Dean's Award for Distinguished Service, the Federation of American Societies for Experimental Biology (FASEB) Special Award for Science Advocacy, and the Friends of the National Institute for Nursing Research's Health Advocacy Award. She is a fellow of the AAAS and a member of the Institute of Medicine and serves as a member of the IOM's Health Science Policy Board and the Clinical Research Roundtable. She earned a BS at Stanford University, an MA at San Francisco State University, and studied advanced management at the University of California, Berkeley.

James B. Wyngaarden, MD, Duke University (NAS, IOM), is Professor Emeritus, Duke University, and currently consults in biotechnology, advising on research agendas as well as strategic planning and organizational start-ups. He previously served as Director of the National Institutes of Health; Associate Director for Life Sciences in the Office of Science and Technology Policy, Executive Office of the President; Director, Human Genome Organization; and Vice Chancellor for Health Affairs at Duke University. He is a member of the National Academy of Sciences and the Institute of Medicine. He earned his MD from University of Michigan Medical School.

Tadataka Yamada, MD GlaxoSmithKline (IOM), is Chairman, Research and Development, Pharmaceuticals at GlaxoSmithKline. Previously, Dr. Yamada was President, SmithKline Beecham Healthcare Services, taking that post in February 1996. He joined SmithKline Beecham as a on-executive member of the Board of Directors in February 1994. He was formerly Chairman of the Department of Internal Medicine at the University of Michigan Medical School and Physician-in-Chief of the University of Michigan Medical Center. Dr Yamada is a Councillor of the Association of American Physicians, past President of the American Gastroenterological Association, and Master of the American College of Physicians. He has been a member of the Board of Directors of the American Board of Internal Medicine and a member at large of the National Board of Medical Examiners. He serves on the Board of Directors of diaDexus and is a Trustee of the Rockefeller Brothers Fund. Dr. Yamada is a graduate of Stanford University with a BA in history. He earned his MD from New York University School of Medicine.